Dictionary of Psychotherapy

This book was created with the aim of providing a comprehensive and easily accessible resource for professionals, students, and anyone interested in psychotherapy. Psychotherapy is a diverse and dynamic field that encompasses a wide range of methods, theories, and techniques aimed at promoting mental health and treating mental disorders.

In recent decades, psychotherapy has made considerable progress and evolved. Numerous approaches and teachings, from classical psychoanalysis to cognitive behavioral therapy to modern mindfulness-based and integrative procedures, reflect the depth and breadth of this field. Each of these methods brings its own concepts and terminologies, which are often specific and sometimes complex.

This dictionary serves as a reference work that explains these terms and puts them in context. It is designed to help you understand definitions and explanations of important concepts, techniques, and theories of psychotherapy. In addition, it contains information on various mental disorders and their treatment approaches.

Our goal is to provide you with a clearly structured and informative reference work that is useful for both the experienced therapist and the newcomer.

We hope that this dictionary will be a useful companion for you in your work and studies and that it will help you to apply and pass on the practice and knowledge of this important field.

TABLE OF CONTENTS

Acceptance and Commitment Therapy (ACT) 13
Acute stress reaction 14
Adjustment disorder 16
Affect 17
Affective disorders 19
Agoraphobia 21
Akinesia 23
Ambitience 24
Amnesia 26
Amplification Plans 27
Anamnesis 30
Anorexia nervosa 31
Anticonvulsants 33
Anti-dementia drugs 34
Antidepressants 36
Anxiety disorder 38
Anxiolytics 40
Anxious-avoidant personality disorder 43
Asperger's syndrome (under autism spectrum disorder) 45
Attachment theory 46
Attention deficit/hyperactivity disorder (ADHD) 48
Autism spectrum disorder 50
Autogenic training 52
Automatisms 54

Avoidance behavior	56
Behavioral therapy	57
Behaviorism	59
Behavioural change	61
Binding Types	63
Binge Eating Disorder	64
Biofeedback	66
Bipolar disorder	68
Bipolar Rapid Cycling	70
Borderline Personality Disorder	72
Bowlby, John	74
Brain function	75
Bridge of Affect	77
Bulimia Nervosa	78
Burnout syndrome	80
Cash register office	82
Catharsis	84
Child and Adolescent Therapy	85
Chronobiology	87
Clinical psychology	88
Cognition	90
Cognitive Behavioral Therapy (CBT)	91
Cognitive dissonance	93
Cognitive restructuring	95
Coma	96
Completion of therapy	98

Conditioning 99
Confabulation 101
Conflict of interests 103
Confrontation 104
Constriction of consciousness 105
Conversational psychotherapy 107
Countertransference 109
Couples Therapy 110
Course of therapy 112
Covering up psychotherapy 113
Crisis intervention 115
Cyclothymia 116
Day clinic 118
Depersonalization 119
Depression 121
Depth Psychology 123
Derealization 124
Diagnosis 125
Diagnostics 127
Dialectical Behavioral Therapy (DBT) 129
Disorientation 130
Dissocial personality disorder 132
Dissociative disorder 134
Disturbance of memory 136
Documentation obligation 137
Dream interpretation 139

Duty to provide information ... 141
Dyslalia/articulation disorder ... 143
Dyssomnias ... 144
Dysthymia ... 146
Eating disorder ... 148
Echopraxia ... 149
Ego disorder ... 151
Elective Mutism ... 153
EMDR (Eye Movement Desensitization and Reprocessing) ... 155
Emotional Intelligence ... 157
Empathy ... 158
Endocrinology ... 160
Enkopresis ... 161
Enuresis ... 162
Epigenetics ... 164
Erickson, Milton ... 166
Existential therapy ... 168
Expansion of consciousness ... 169
Exposure method ... 171
Expressive speech disorder ... 173
Family constellation ... 175
Family history ... 176
Family Therapy ... 178
Fight-or-flight ... 179
Flow ... 181

Framing 182
Freud, Sigmund 184
Further education 186
Generalized anxiety disorder 187
Geriatric Psychotherapy 189
Gestalt therapy 191
Group therapy 193
Habituation 194
Hallucinations 196
Heller's dementia 197
Histrionic personality disorder 199
Holy Seven (after Alexanders) 201
Humanistic Therapy 203
Hyperkinesia 205
Hypersomnia 206
Hypnotherapy 208
Hypochondriacal disorder 210
I/Superego 211
ICD-10 214
Illusory misjudgement 215
Imagination 216
Immune system and psyche 218
Impulse control disorders 220
Individual therapy 221
Inner child 223
Inpatient therapy 225

Insomnia/hyposomnia ... 226
Intellectual disability/oligophrenia ... 228
Interpersonal Therapy (IPT) ... 230
Intervention ... 232
Logorrhea ... 234
Mania ... 236
Mourning ... 237
Mutism ... 239
Narcissistic personality disorder ... 241
Negative symptoms ... 242
Neologisms ... 244
Neuroasthenia (also known as fatigue syndrome) ... 245
Neuroplasticity ... 247
Neurosis ... 249
Neurotransmitter ... 250
OCD ... 252
Online therapy ... 254
Orthorexia ... 256
Outpatient therapy ... 257
Paramnesia ... 259
Paranoid personality disorder ... 260
Parasomnias ... 262
Perception disorder (syn.: apperception) ... 264
Personal history ... 266
Personality disorder ... 267
Phobia ... 269

- Pica in childhood 271
- Pledge of secrecy 272
- Positive symptoms 274
- Post-traumatic stress disorder (PTSD) 275
- Pre-suicidal syndrome 277
- Professional Code of Conduct 279
- Professional ethics 280
- Professional indemnity 282
- Projection 283
- Psychiatric emergencies 285
- Psychoanalysis 287
- Psychodynamic therapy 289
- Psychoeducation 291
- Psychosomatics 292
- Psychotherapy 294
- Reactive attachment disorder of childhood 296
- Receptive speech disorder 298
- Reframing 300
- Relapse prevention 301
- Resilience 303
- Resistance 304
- Rett syndrome 306
- Revealing psychotherapy 307
- Roleplaying game 309
- Rorschach Test 310
- Rumble 312

Schema therapy 314
Schizoid personality disorder 316
Schizophrenia 318
Self-instruction training 320
Sense of coherence 321
Sensory illusions or perceptual illusions 323
Sexual dysfunction 325
Sleep disorder 327
Sleep phases 328
Social history 330
Social phobia 332
Social Skills Training 334
Somatization disorder 336
Somatoform autonomic dysfunction 337
Somatoform disorder 339
Somnambulism 341
Somnolence 342
Sopor 344
Stereotypical movement disorder 345
Stress 347
Stress management training 349
Stress reaction 351
Stupor 352
Suicidal tendencies according to Pöldinger 354
Suicide 356
Supervision 357

Supervisor/Supervisor 359
Systemic therapy 360
Therapeutic Alliance 363
Therapeutic limits 364
Therapeutic relationship 366
Therapist's self-care 368
Therapy goals 370
Thinking disorders 371
Tick disorders 373
Transactional analysis 374
Transfer 377
Trauma therapy 378
Treatment 380
Treatment contract 382
Unconsciousness 383
Vulnerability 385

Acceptance and Commitment Therapy (ACT)

Acceptance and Commitment Therapy (ACT) is a form of cognitive behavioral therapy that focuses on promoting psychological flexibility. Developed by Steven C. Hayes and his colleagues in the 1980s, ACT is based on the assumption that many mental health problems arise from trying to avoid or control unpleasant thoughts and feelings.

A central concept in ACT is **acceptance**. This involves acknowledging unpleasant thoughts and feelings and giving them space instead of fighting them or avoiding them. Acceptance reduces resistance to one's own experience and enables a more open approach to difficult emotions.

ACT works with **mindfulness techniques** that aim to help clients stay in the present moment and perceive their experiences without judgment. This mindfulness is crucial for developing acceptance, as it allows clients to observe their thoughts and feelings without being overwhelmed by them.

Another important element of ACT is **commitment**, i.e. committing to personal values and acting in accordance with these values. ACT helps clients identify their most fundamental beliefs and goals and encourages them to actively take steps toward those values, even if unpleasant thoughts and feelings arise in the process.

To do this, ACT uses a variety of **metaphorical exercises** and **experiential exercises** to support clients in changing their relationship with their thoughts and feelings. One example is the concept of "entangled thinking," where clients learn how to get caught up in thought loops and what ways there are to distance themselves from them.

Another significant concept is **cognitive defusion**, which involves reducing the influence of thoughts by recognizing them as simple mental events, rather than true or meaningful. Clients practice observing and accepting their thoughts, rather than blindly following them or identifying with them.

ACT also emphasizes **personal responsibility** and the **active decision** to live a values-based life. Clients are encouraged to identify concrete, actionable steps that will help them put their values into action. This can be supported by goal setting and the development of action plans.

By integrating elements of acceptance and mindfulness with behaviour change techniques, ACT aims to expand clients' scope of action and help them live more fulfilling and meaningful lives, despite the inevitable challenges and pains of the human condition.

Acute stress reaction

The Acute Stress Response describes a temporary mental disorder that occurs as a direct result of extraordinary physical or mental stress. This reaction occurs immediately after an extremely stressful or traumatic event and is temporary, often lasting from a few minutes to a few days. As a rule, the symptoms subside after a short time, but in some cases the stress reaction can turn into a chronic disorder.

A central feature of the acute stress reaction is the occurrence of significant impairments in the emotional and cognitive areas, which can manifest themselves in mild to severe symptoms. Typical symptoms are intense fear, panic, despair, helplessness and a general overwhelm of the individual. Physically, sweating, palpitations, tremors and shortness of breath can occur. Cognitively, it can lead to difficulties in concentration, perceptual distortions and memory problems.

Theoretically, it is assumed that the acute stress reaction serves as a natural, evolutionary reaction to extreme stressors. It represents a kind of psychological emergency mode that is intended to enable the affected person to react quickly and efficiently to life-threatening situations. This reaction can be seen as an impetus for fight or flight behavior, whereby the body and mind are trimmed to peak performance in order to cope with the threatening situation.

In psychotherapeutic practice, it is important to stabilize the affected person through appropriate interventions and to alleviate the symptoms. To do this, it can be helpful to actively listen to those affected, to reassure them and to convey to them that their reactions are a normal reaction to an extraordinary situation. Psychotherapeutic measures can include relaxation techniques, cognitive restructuring and support in processing the trauma. The aim is to restore self-efficacy and a sense of control in the affected person.

Pharmacological measures can also be considered, especially if anxiety and sleep disorders dominate. Benzodiazepines or other anxiolytic drugs can be used for a short time, although the risk of developing dependence must always be taken into account.

In the long term, it is relevant for those affected to develop strategies to better cope with future stress. Techniques for stress management, psychoeducation and, if necessary, further trauma therapy can contribute to this. Each treatment should be individually adapted to the needs of the affected person and support him or her in the best possible way in his process of processing and healing.

Adjustment disorder

Adjustment disorder is a mental illness that arises when a person reacts to a significant change or stressful life events with inappropriate and persistent emotional or behavioral reactions. These events can be varied, from losses such as the death of a loved one or separation, to major changes such as moving or changing jobs, to ongoing stresses such as chronic illness or financial problems.

Clinically, an adjustment disorder manifests itself through symptoms that can range from anxiety, depression and irritability to social withdrawal and disturbed everyday behavior. These symptoms appear within three months of the triggering event and cause significant stress or impairment in the social, occupational, or other important functional areas of the affected person.

A characteristic feature is that the symptoms go beyond what might be expected given the severity and nature of the stressful event. For example, after a divorce, a person might have a significantly stronger and long-lasting depressive reaction than other people in similar situations would.

The diagnosis of adjustment disorder requires that the symptoms cannot be better explained by another mental disorder such as major depression or an anxiety disorder. It is also important to distinguish that the reactions do not fall within the range of a normal grief reaction.

Therapeutically, adjustment disorder can be accompanied by various approaches. Psychotherapeutic interventions such as cognitive behavioral therapy (CBT) can help identify and change maladaptive patterns of thought and behavior. Likewise, the support of a social network can play a significant role and promote the adaptation process.

Drug treatment approaches can be used as a supplement, especially if the emotional symptoms are particularly severe and significantly impair the functioning of the affected person. For example, antidepressants or anxiolytic medications can provide short-term relief.

The prognosis of adjustment disorder is generally good, especially if professional help is sought early. Symptoms typically subside within a few months after the affected person has begun to deal with or cope with the new life situation. However, untreated adjustment disorders can increase the risk of developing more serious mental illnesses, which is why proper diagnosis and treatment are crucial.

Affect

The term "affect" refers to a short-term, intense emotional state, which is usually spontaneous and accompanied by a high physiological and expressive component. Affects can be triggered by internal or external stimuli and are of shorter duration compared to emotions or moods. While emotions represent more comprehensive psychological states and moods are longer-lasting emotional states, affects are often abrupt and characterized by strong intensity.

Affects can be initiated by various causes, including immediate sensory impressions, memories, or mental associations. They affect the entire organism and manifest themselves both physiologically and behavioristically. Physiologically, changes in the cardiovascular system, breathing and muscle tension are typical. These somatic reactions prepare the body for rapid adaptation, which is evolutionary and can ensure survival in dangerous situations.

Behavioristically, affects express themselves through clearly visible changes in expressive behavior, such as body language, facial expressions and gestures. A person in the affect can perform uncontrolled actions that are often perceived as irrational or disproportionate in retrospect. Therefore, the regulation of affects plays an important role in the treatment of mental disorders.

In a therapeutic context, special attention is paid to the way in which a client experiences, expresses and regulates affects. An improperly discharged affect can contribute to interpersonal conflicts, social isolation or self-harming behaviour. Talk therapies, behavioral therapies and other methods aim to provide clients with tools to better deal with spontaneously occurring, intense emotional states.

In addition, affects are of particular interest in psychodynamic therapy. In this approach, the expression and repression of affects is considered essential for the emergence of psychological conflicts. Through the therapeutic process, an attempt is made to uncover the repressed affects and to make them consciously tangible in order to lead the client to a deeper understanding of his emotions and behavior.

Affective disorders

Affective disorders are a category of mental illnesses that are primarily characterized by significant changes in mood and emotions. These disorders have a significant impact on a person's emotional experience and behavior. The main categories of mood disorders include depressive disorder, bipolar disorder, and seasonal affective disorder.

Depressive disorders

Depressive disorders are characterized by persistent feelings of deep sadness, hopelessness and anhedonia, i.e. the loss of the ability to feel joy. Symptoms also include sleep disturbances, changes in appetite, concentration problems and reduced energy. In severe cases, suicidal thoughts can occur.

Bipolar disorder

Bipolar disorder is characterized by extreme mood swings that alternate between manic and depressive episodes. Manic episodes include increased energy, euphoria, irritability, decreased need for sleep, and impulsive behavior. Depressive episodes in this context are similar to the symptoms of major depressive disorder.

Seasonal Affective Disorder (SAD)

This form of affective disorder is closely linked to the seasons, usually occurring during the winter months when daylight is reduced. Those affected experience symptoms of depression that begin in the months with less light and subside in the spring and summer months.

Causes

The causes of mood disorders are complex and multifactorial. Neurobiological aspects such as neurotransmitter imbalances, genetic predispositions, hormonal fluctuations and structural or functional brain changes may play a role. Environmental factors such as traumatic events, chronic stress, and sociocultural context also contribute.

Treatment

Treatment of mood disorders often involves a combination of pharmacological and psychotherapeutic approaches. Antidepressants, mood stabilizers, and antipsychotics can be used to relieve symptoms. Psychotherapeutic interventions such as cognitive behavioral therapy (CBT), interpersonal therapy (IPT), and mindfulness-based therapies have been shown to be effective.

Importance in psychotherapy

In psychotherapeutic practice, understanding affective disorders is essential in order to develop targeted and individualized treatment plans. Early intervention can have a positive influence on the course of the disease and reduce the risk of serious complications. Regular supervision and further training are necessary to maintain and expand diagnostic and therapeutic skills.

Mood disorders are widespread and affect people of all ages and social classes. Their treatment requires a deep understanding of both the biological basis and the individual and social context of those affected.

Agoraphobia

Agoraphobia is a complex anxiety disorder characterized by persistent and intense fear of situations or places where escape could be difficult or embarrassing, or where help would not be available in the event of panic symptoms. The term comes from the Greek and literally means "fear of the marketplace", alluding to the classic, spacious squares that people with this disorder often avoid.

This fear is not limited to open spaces, but can include numerous situations such as staying in crowds, leaving the house alone, using public transport, standing or waiting in a queue, or other environments that are perceived as unsafe.

The symptoms of agoraphobia can vary, but often affected people experience physical symptoms such as palpitations, dizziness, nausea, tremors, and sweating. These symptoms are often signs of a panic attack, which can occur in the feared situations. A panic attack is a sudden episode of intense anxiety that causes significant physical and emotional discomfort.

Out of the fear of these symptoms, those affected develop avoidance strategies. These can range from being accompanied by trusted people to complete isolation in one's own home. Such behaviors can have a massive impact on everyday life and often lead to social isolation, professional difficulties and a poorer quality of life.

The development of agoraphobia can be multifactorial. Genetic predispositions, traumatic experiences, certain personality traits and dysfunctional thought patterns can contribute to the development of this anxiety disorder. In particular, fear of losing control and experiencing traumatic events in the past often play a significant role.

In the treatment of agoraphobia, cognitive behavioral therapies are in the foreground. These aim to identify and gradually modify irrational fears and avoidance behaviors. A central component is exposure therapy, in which those affected face the feared situations under guidance and in small steps. In the process, they learn to deal with their anxiety symptoms and learn that the feared catastrophes usually do not occur.

In addition, drug treatments, such as taking antidepressants or benzodiazepines, can be considered, especially if the symptoms are severe. Support through mindfulness training and relaxation techniques can also be helpful in lowering general anxiety levels and improving quality of life.

The prognosis of agoraphobia varies from person to person, but with appropriate therapeutic support, many sufferers can achieve a significant improvement in their lifestyle and a reduction in anxiety symptoms.

Akinesia

Akinese is a medical term that comes from the Greek and translates as "motionlessness". In psychotherapy and medical circles, Akinese describes the phenomenon of limited or absent motor activity. It is a movement disorder in which the affected person has considerable difficulty initiating or performing movements.

Akinesis is common in neurological and psychiatric disorders, especially Parkinson's disease, where it is one of the main symptoms. Patients with akinesis show reduced spontaneous motor function and experience difficulty performing voluntary movements. This can be noticeable in everyday life through slow, stiff or not performed movements at all. Getting up from a chair, starting a walk, or even simply reaching for an object can become major challenges.

Akinesis is also a relevant symptom in psychiatry, for example in certain forms of schizophrenia or when taking antipsychotics, especially so-called typical neuroleptics. As a side effect, these drugs can cause a kind of drug-induced Parkinson's symptoms, which also includes akinesis.

The neurobiological basis of akinesis is complex and involves dysfunctions in different parts of the brain, especially in the area of the basal ganglia, which are responsible for regulating and coordinating movements. Dopamine deficiency in the striatum, a part of the basal ganglia, is often thought to be the immediate cause of movement inhibition, which explains akinesis in Parkinson's patients.

Therapeutically, akinesis is treated differently depending on the underlying cause. In Parkinson's patients, dopaminergic drugs are often used to compensate for the lack of dopamine in the brain. In drug-induced akinesis, medication adjustment or switching to atypical antipsychotics, which have a lower risk of such side effects, may be considered.

In a psychosocial context, akinesis can have significant consequences for the everyday life and quality of life of those affected. Limited mobility can lead to social isolation, as the patient may avoid activities that they used to enjoy. Therefore, in psychotherapeutic work, it is important not only to see akinesis as an isolated physical symptom, but also to consider its influence on emotional and social health. Supportive measures such as physiotherapy, occupational therapy and social care can be helpful in increasing patients' quality of life and enabling them to live as independently as possible.

Accompaniment by a therapist who understands the patient's psychosocial needs is crucial to develop appropriate coping strategies and encourage the patient to actively participate in life despite limitations.

Ambitience

In psychotherapy, ambitencing refers to a phenomenon in which an individual simultaneously feels opposing impulses, desires or tendencies and has difficulty deciding between them. This concept is often found in the context of mental conflicts and inner turmoil and is particularly relevant when working with clients who suffer from ambivalent feelings.

Ambitency can manifest itself in various areas of life, including choices, relationships, and personal goals. For example, a person might feel both the urge to seek a close relationship with another person and at the same time be afraid of closeness and avoid that relationship. These conflicting impulses can lead to significant emotional distress as the individual fails to find clear direction and feels torn.

In therapeutic practice, it is of great importance to recognize and understand the ambitencies of a client. These dual tendencies can result from previous experiences, unresolved inner conflicts, or deep-rooted fears. A deep understanding of these opposing impulses can help to uncover the underlying psychological mechanisms and develop specific intervention strategies.

Working with ambitency often requires the use of various therapeutic techniques, such as the exploration of thoughts and feelings, the use of imagination exercises or the conduct of an inner dialogue. The aim is to help the client identify the sources of inner conflicts, develop a deeper understanding of themselves and develop strategies to deal with these contradictory tendencies.

Successfully dealing with ambitency can make a significant contribution to reducing stress and emotional strain. It allows the client to make clearer decisions and develop a more coherent self-image. In the long term, this can lead to an improved quality of life and more stable interpersonal relationships.

Amnesia

Amnesia refers to a partial or complete loss of memory. It can be the result of physical trauma, psychological stress or neurodegenerative processes and affects different types of memories, including episodic, semantic and procedural memory content.

One of the typical classifications of amnesia is based on temporal criteria: retrograde amnesia, in which the patient can no longer remember events that occurred before the triggering event, and anterograde amnesia, in which the ability to form new memories is impaired. There are cases in which both forms occur simultaneously, which significantly affects the entire memory.

Clinically, a distinction is also made between psychogenic and organic amnesia. Psychogenic amnesia, also known as dissociative amnesia, is usually triggered by psychological trauma or severe emotional conflicts. It often occurs suddenly and can selectively affect certain periods of time or events. In contrast, organic amnesia results from physical causes such as traumatic brain injury, brain infections or neurodegenerative diseases such as Alzheimer's. This form often has a gradual onset and progressive deterioration.

The effects of amnesia on the patient's everyday life vary greatly depending on the extent and type of memory loss. In many cases, short-term memory is preserved, while long-term memory is severely impaired or vice versa. Affected individuals may have difficulty remembering everyday routines or storing new information, which can significantly affect their ability to be independent and their quality of life.

Therapeutic approaches to the treatment of amnesia are diverse and often interdisciplinary. In psychotherapeutic treatment, the primary attempt is to make repressed memories and emotions accessible through techniques such as hypnosis or cognitive behavioral therapy. The processing and integration of traumatic experiences also plays a central role.

In the case of organic amnesia, neurorehabilitative measures, memory training and pharmacological interventions can be used to support and improve cognitive function. In any case, the treatment requires an individual and coordinated approach, as the specific triggers and effects of amnesia are different for each affected person.

Psychotherapists work closely with neurologists and other specialists to make a comprehensive diagnosis and develop appropriate treatment strategies. Through a precise medical history and targeted psychometric tests, the extent and type of amnesia can be recorded in detail.

Amplification Plans

Reinforcement plans are structured programs or systematic approaches that are used in behavior modification to reinforce or promote certain behaviors. They are based on the principles of operant conditioning, a form of learning in which behavior is influenced by consequences. Reinforcement plans are a central element in many psychotherapeutic approaches, especially in behavioral and behavioral therapy.

In operant conditioning, the likelihood of behavior is increased by the introduction of reinforcers. An amplifier is a stimulus that, when presented after a behavior, increases the future likelihood of that behavior occurring. Amplifiers can be positive or negative. Positive reinforcers are rewards or pleasant stimuli that follow a behavior, while negative reinforcers are unpleasant stimuli that are removed or diminished by a behavior.

Amplification plans can be divided into different types that target how and when amplifiers are presented to maintain the desired behavior:

1. Continuous Reinforcement:

In this plan, any occurrence of the desired behavior is reinforced. This is especially effective when a behavior is first learned. However, it is not very practical for long-term use, as the amplification must be constant, and saturation can quickly occur, at which the enhancer loses its effectiveness.

2. Intermittent reinforcement:

Here, the behavior is only occasionally reinforced, making it more resistant to extinction (the disappearance of behavior). Intermittent amplification can be further classified into different subtypes:

- **Fixed Interval:** Gain is given after a fixed period of time, once the behavior has occurred. For example, every ten minutes, the behavior is reinforced if it occurred within those ten minutes.
- **Variable Interval:** The amount of time between amplifications varies unpredictably,

but on average over a period of time. This creates constant and sustained behavior.
- **Fixed ratio:** Reinforcement occurs after a fixed number of reactions. For example, reinforcement is given after every fifth reaction.
- **Variable Ratio:** The number of reactions required to obtain reinforcement varies, resulting in a high and steady reaction pattern. Gambling machines are a typical example of variable quotient.

3. **Aversion control:**

In this case, unpleasant stimulus is removed when the desired behavior is shown. This is a form of negative reinforcement and can be effective in reinforcing behavior by providing relief.

The choice of reinforcement plan depends on several factors, including the type of behavior to be modified, the client's age and stage of development, and the specific goals of the therapy. A carefully thought-out reinforcement plan can help to achieve sustainable behavioral changes and efficiently achieve the therapeutic goals. Reinforcement schedules need to be reviewed and adjusted regularly to maximize their effectiveness and ensure that they meet the client's needs.

Anamnesis

In psychotherapy, the term "anamnesis" refers to the systematic process of collecting a patient's medical history. This process is a fundamental part of therapeutic work, as it provides the basis for diagnosis, treatment planning and the therapeutic course.

The anamnesis usually begins with the first contact with the patient and can take place in one or more detailed discussions. The therapist collects information on various areas of the patient's life, including medical, psychological, social and family backgrounds.

A central part of the anamnesis is the symptom anamnesis, in which the therapist asks for detailed information about the patient's current complaints. The type, duration, intensity, and course of the symptoms are described in detail. Possible triggers and alleviating factors are also discussed.

Another important area is the biographical anamnesis. Here, the patient's life history is recorded, including childhood, school years, professional development and family situation. Particularly important are previous traumatic events or formative experiences that could influence the current psychological state.

In the medical anamnesis, all relevant physical illnesses and medical treatments are asked. These include past surgeries, chronic illnesses, current medications and any known allergies. This information is crucial in order to be able to identify and rule out possible somatic causes of psychological symptoms.

The social anamnesis includes questions about relationship status, social network, professional and financial situations, as well as leisure activities and hobbies. Information about current stress factors or conflicts in the patient's social environment is also collected and analyzed.

The family history aims to inquire about the occurrence of mental and somatic illnesses within the family, as genetic and familial predispositions can play an important role. It also examines family structures and dynamics that may have an impact on the patient's mental health.

The psychodynamic part of the anamnesis refers to inner conflicts, defense mechanisms and relationship patterns. The therapist examines here which unconscious processes may contribute to the development and maintenance of the symptoms.

The anamnesis is not static, but a dynamic process that can be supplemented and updated again and again in the course of therapy. The information obtained provides a rich basis for the development of a comprehensive understanding of the patient and his personal history, which is essential for the tailor-made planning and implementation of the therapy.

Anorexia nervosa

Anorexia nervosa is a serious eating disorder characterized by an intense desire for weight loss and extreme food reduction. This disorder is characterized by a deep-rooted fear of gaining weight, although affected people are often already significantly underweight. The perception of one's own body is strongly distorted; those affected continue to see themselves as "too fat", even if they are objectively severely malnourished.

The disease occurs predominantly in adolescents and young adults and affects women more often than men. Typical symptoms include extreme calorie restriction, excessive exercise, monitoring one's own weight, and the use of laxative medications or diuretics. Often, sufferers skip meals or eat only very small amounts of "safe" foods that are considered non-fattening.

The physiological consequences of anorexia nervosa are serious. Insufficient nutrient intake leads to a variety of health problems such as cardiac arrhythmias, osteoporosis, anemia, and a weakened immune system. Other complications can include hair loss, dry skin, kidney failure, and electrolyte imbalances. In extreme cases, this disorder can be fatal.

Psychological symptoms of this condition include severely decreased self-esteem, obsessive thoughts about food and weight, and depression and anxiety. Those affected often isolate themselves socially and avoid situations that focus on food or the body in order to avoid criticism or remarks about their eating habits and weight.

The treatment of anorexia nervosa requires a multimodal approach. This includes psychotherapeutic support, medical monitoring and, in many cases, nutritional counselling. Cognitive behavioral therapy (CBT) has been shown to be effective in changing underlying dysfunctional beliefs about food, weight, and self-worth. Family-based therapy can also be helpful, especially in younger patients, to address family dynamics and provide support in the home setting.

Early diagnosis and therapy are crucial for positive treatment prognosis. Due to the complex nature of this disorder, which affects psychological, social and physical aspects, an interdisciplinary treatment team is often required to create the best possible individual treatment plan.

Anticonvulsants

Anticonvulsants are drugs that are primarily used to treat and control seizure disorders such as epilepsy. These drugs aim to regulate the excessive neuronal activity in the brain that is responsible for causing seizures. However, the effectiveness of anticonvulsants in stabilizing electrical activity in the brain also makes them relevant and beneficial for various mental disorders.

In addition to their use in epilepsy treatment, anticonvulsants are used in psychotherapy and psychiatry to stabilize mood and in the therapy of mood disorders. In bipolar disorder, they mainly help to mitigate or prevent manic and hypomanic episodes by dampening the excitability of the neural network. Examples of commonly used anticonvulsants in this context are valproic acid, carbamazepine and lamotrigine. These substances have different mechanisms of action, ranging from inhibiting voltage-gated sodium channels to increasing gamma-aminobutyric acid (GABA) function, an important inhibitory neurotransmitter.

In addition, anticonvulsants have been found useful in treating anxiety disorders. Their anxiolytic properties are due to the ability to reduce neuronal overexcitation, which contributes to an overall calming of the CNS (central nervous system). In some cases, anticonvulsants can also be used as adjunctive therapy in patients who do not respond adequately to classic antidepressant or anxiolytic drugs.

Because anticonvulsants have a wide range of neurobiological effects, clinical applications go beyond traditional use. They are also used in the treatment of neuropathic pain and even in some cases of borderline personality disorder due to their neuroprotective properties.

As with all medications, careful control and adjustment by a specialist is necessary to achieve optimal therapeutic results while minimizing side effects. Common side effects include sedation, weight gain, dizziness, and cognitive impairment. Particular attention should be paid to the potential risk of liver toxicity or haematological disorders with long-term use.

Anti-dementia drugs

Anti-dementia drugs are drug therapies that have been specially developed to alleviate the symptoms of dementia and slow down the progression of the disease. Dementias, such as Alzheimer's disease or vascular dementia, are characterized by progressive loss of cognitive function, including memory, decision-making, and orientation. These drugs target precisely these problem areas to enable those affected to stay longer in their familiar environment and improve their quality of life.

The pharmacological basis of anti-dementia drugs can be divided into two main categories: cholinesterase inhibitors and NMDA receptor antagonists.

Cholinesterase inhibitors: These substances, such as donepezil, rivastigmine, and galantamine, work by inhibiting the enzyme acetylcholinesterase. This enzyme is responsible for the breakdown of acetylcholine in the brain. By inhibiting degradation, more acetylcholine remains available in the synaptic cleft, which improves communication between nerve cells. This enhancement of cholinergic transmission can relieve the symptoms of memory loss and cognitive impairment, at least temporarily.

NMDA receptor antagonists: A well-known representative of this group is memantine. NMDA receptors are binding sites for the neurotransmitter glutamate, which plays a key role in excitatory synaptic transmissions in the brain. In pathological processes of dementia, overactivation of these receptors can lead to neuronal damage and apoptosis. Memantine regulates this overactivation by blocking the NMDA receptor without completely inhibiting normal neuronal transmission, which can potentially slow down the loss of nerve cells.

Furthermore, there are also non-pharmacological approaches that are used in addition to drug treatment and can make a significant contribution to improving quality of life. These include cognitive training programs, behavioral therapy interventions and targeted social and physical activation of those affected.

Although antidementia drugs are not able to cure the disease or stop the progression of the disease for good, they do help slow progression and stabilize cognitive performance. This can mean that patients are able to manage everyday activities independently for longer. It also allows for a slightly longer period of autonomy and self-determination, which can be very significant for both those affected and their relatives.

However, the efficacy and tolerability of these drugs varies widely between individuals, and not every patient responds equally well to treatment. Therefore, an individual adaptation of the drug therapy as well as regular monitoring and adjustment by the attending physician is essential.

Antidepressants

Antidepressants are a class of medications that are primarily used to treat depressive disorders. They are also used in the therapy of anxiety disorders, obsessive-compulsive disorder, post-traumatic stress disorder and various other psychological and somatic conditions. These drugs aim to regulate the chemical balance in the brain, especially in relation to neurotransmitters such as serotonin, norepinephrine, and dopamine, which are believed to play an essential role in mood control and emotional stability.

There are several main types of antidepressants, which differ in their chemical structure and mode of action:

1. **Selective serotonin reuptake inhibitors (SSRIs):**

SSRIs such as fluoxetine, paroxetine, and sertraline block the reuptake of serotonin into the presynaptic nerve cells, resulting in increased availability of this neurotransmitter in the synaptic cleft. This can promote mood enhancement and anxiety relief. SSRIs are often the preferred choice in the initial treatment of depression due to their comparatively favorable side effect profile and effectiveness.

2. Serotonin-norepinephrine reuptake inhibitors (SNRIs):

SNRIs such as venlafaxine and duloxetine block the reuptake of both serotonin and norepinephrine. This dual mode of action may be helpful for patients for whom SSRI medications have not been sufficiently effective. However, SNRIs can also have a different side effect profile.

3. Tricyclic antidepressants (TCAs):

TCAs such as amitriptyline and clomipramine block the reuptake of serotonin and norepinephrine, but less selectively than SSRIs and SNRIs. They also act on a variety of other receptors in the brain, which enhances their effectiveness, but also increases the likelihood of side effects such as dry mouth, sedation, and weight gain. They are often used as a second or third choice, especially in patients with chronic or therapy-resistant depression.

4. Monoamine oxidase inhibitors (MAOIs):

MAOIs such as tranylcypromine and phenelzine inhibit the activity of the enzyme monoamine oxidase, which is responsible for the breakdown of monoamines such as serotonin, norepinephrine and dopamine. Despite their potential effectiveness in certain forms of depression, MAOIs are rarely used as first-line therapy due to their serious interactions with certain foods and other medications.

5. Atypical antidepressants:

This group includes medications that do not fall into the above categories, such as bupropion and mirtazapine. Bupropion acts primarily on the reuptake of dopamine and norepinephrine, while mirtazapine exerts its effect by blocking specific serotonin and norepinephrine receptors. Atypical antidepressants can be a valuable treatment option, especially for patients who do not respond to or tolerate other medications.

Side effects of antidepressants can be varied, ranging from mild discomfort such as nausea and insomnia to more serious side effects such as sexual dysfunction or increased risk of suicide, especially in the first few weeks of treatment or in younger patients. It is therefore crucial to monitor patients closely during the initial phase of treatment.

The choice of the specific antidepressant depends on various factors, including the individual course of symptoms, previous pharmacological experience, the side effect profile and concomitant physical illnesses of the patient. Careful consideration and possibly a time-limited trial-and-error approach is often required to find the most appropriate drug and dose for each patient.

Finally, it should be noted that antidepressants are often used in combination with psychotherapeutic procedures such as cognitive behavioral therapy (CBT). These integrative approaches have proven to be particularly effective as they address both the chemical and psychological dimensions of depression and related disorders.

Anxiety disorder

Anxiety disorder refers to a mental illness in which people are affected by excessive anxiety and fear, which are often disproportionate to the actual threat. This condition is characterized by persistent or recurrent anxiety that can significantly limit everyday life.

There are several forms of anxiety disorders, including generalized anxiety disorder (GAD), panic disorder, specific phobias, social anxiety disorder (social phobia), and agoraphobia. These different forms manifest themselves in specific symptoms and behavioral patterns.

Generalized anxiety disorder (GAD) focuses on persistent and excessive worry that is not limited to a specific situation. Sufferers often experience physical symptoms such as muscle tension, sleep problems, and irritability, which go hand in hand with constant worry.

Panic disorder is characterized by recurrent, sudden panic attacks that cause intense anxiety and severe physical symptoms such as palpitations, dizziness and shortness of breath. These attacks often occur without warning and can cause sufferers to avoid certain situations or places for fear of experiencing another attack.

Specific phobias are strong, irrational fears of certain objects or situations, such as heights, spiders or air travel. These fears often lead to avoidance behavior, which can have a strong influence on the everyday life of those affected.

Social anxiety disorder is an intense fear of social situations in which sufferers fear negative evaluations by others. This anxiety can lead them to avoid social interactions or experience extreme tension in social contexts. This can significantly restrict professional and private life.

Agoraphobia refers to the fear of situations where escape would be difficult or helpless, such as in crowds or wide open spaces. This fear can result in far-reaching avoidance patterns that severely restrict those affected in their freedom of movement.

The causes of anxiety disorders are diverse and include genetic factors, biochemical imbalances, traumatic experiences, and learned behavioral patterns. There are often comorbidities with other mental illnesses such as depression or addictions.

Treatment for anxiety disorders can include a variety of approaches. Cognitive behavioral therapy (CBT) is an established method that aims to recognize and change dysfunctional patterns of thought and behavior. Exposure therapy, a component of CBT, helps those affected to gradually face and cope with their fears.

Drug therapies, especially antidepressants and anxiolytics, can also be used to treat anxiety disorders. In addition, relaxation techniques, mindfulness training and physical activity can be supportive measures that can alleviate the symptoms.

Anxiolytics

Anxiolytics, also known as anxiety relievers or anxiolytic drugs, are a class of psychotropic drugs that are primarily used to treat anxiety and its side effects. These pharmacological substances act on the central nervous system (CNS) and reduce symptoms of anxiety, tension and agitation without having the sedative effect of sleeping pills, at least in therapeutic dosages.

Mechanisms

Most anxiolytics work by modulating neurotransmitters in the brain, especially the gamma-aminobutyric acid (GABA) system. GABA is an inhibitory neurotransmitter that decreases neuronal excitability in the CNS. Anxiolytics such as benzodiazepines promote the effect of GABA by binding to specific receptors (GABA_A receptors) and enhancing their inhibitory effects. This pharmacological enhancement of the GABA system results in a calming and anxiolytic effect.

Categories and examples

Benzodiazepines: This is the most commonly prescribed class of anxiolytics. Well-known examples are diazepam (Valium), lorazepam (Ativan), and alprazolam (Xanax). They provide quick relief from anxiety and are especially effective for acute anxiety or panic attacks. However, their use should be short-term and under strict medical supervision, as dependence and tolerance can develop with prolonged use.

Serotonin reuptake inhibitors (SSRIs) and serotonin-norepinephrine reuptake inhibitors (SNRIs): These classes of antidepressants, which include medications such as fluoxetine (Prozac), sertraline (Zoloft), and venlafaxine (Effexor), are also commonly used to treat anxiety disorders. Their mechanism of action includes inhibiting the reuptake of serotonin and norepinephrine, which increases the concentration of these neurotransmitters in the synaptic cleft and thereby has a mood-enhancing and anti-anxiety effect. Compared to benzodiazepines, SSRIs and SNRIs act less quickly, but more sustainably and without the risk of rapid dependence development.

Buspirone: Another representative of the anxiolytics, which is mainly used for generalized anxiety disorder. It acts as a partial agonist at the serotonin 5-HT1A receptor and has no sedative effect. The effect sets in rather slowly, often only after several weeks of continuous use.

Indications

Anxiolytics are prescribed for various forms of anxiety disorders, including:

- Generalized anxiety disorder (GAD)
- Social anxiety disorder (SAD)
- Panic disorder
- Post-traumatic stress disorder (PTSD)
- Obsessive-Compulsive Disorder (OCD)

Anxiolytics are also used in the treatment of psychosomatic illnesses, in which anxiety plays an essential role.

Side effects and risks

While anxiolytics are often indispensable aids in anxiety therapy, they can also cause side effects. These include drowsiness, sedation, dizziness, coordination disorders and the risk of developing dependence (especially with benzodiazepines). Withdrawal symptoms may occur if you stop it suddenly.

When taking SSRIs and SNRIs, initially increased feelings of anxiety often occur, which subside after a few weeks. Other side effects may include nausea, trouble sleeping, and sexual dysfunction.

Deployment and monitoring

The therapeutic goal in the use of anxiolytics is to alleviate symptoms and allow the affected person to participate in psychotherapeutic interventions or regain everyday functions. Continuous monitoring by the attending physician or psychotherapist is necessary to adjust the dosage and detect any side effects at an early stage.

In psychotherapeutic practice, drug treatment should always be integrated into a comprehensive treatment program that includes psychotherapeutic techniques such as cognitive behavioral therapy (CBT), exposure techniques, and relaxation techniques.

Anxious-avoidant personality disorder

Anxious-avoidant personality disorder (APD) is a pervasive mental disorder characterized by an overwhelming sense of social incompetence, inferiority, and extreme sensitivity to negative evaluation. This disorder often begins in early adulthood and manifests itself in different situations and contexts of a person's life.

People with APPs have a persistent and widespread fear of being rejected, criticized, or judged negatively. They show impressive restraint in social interactions and tend to withdraw from social, professional, or other activities where they could potentially connect with others. This often leads to considerable social isolation. Despite their desire for closer relationships and social bonds, they prefer to stay alone for fear of exposure or rejection.

A central feature of the ÄVPS is the highly disadvantaged self-image. Those affected often see themselves as socially awkward, uninteresting or inferior compared to others. This negative self-perception is reinforced by past experiences of rejection or criticism, creating a vicious cycle: out of fear of rejection, they avoid social interactions, which in turn leads to fewer opportunities to gain positive social experiences and improve self-image.

Individuals with ÄVPS are overly wary of potential signs of rejection or criticism. They often mistakenly interpret neutral or even positive social cues as negative and react to them with even greater restraint and avoidance. This increases isolation and prevents the build-up of self-confidence in social situations.

In therapeutic contexts, working with patients with APPs is challenging, as their deep-rooted fear of criticism and rejection is often present to the therapist. A step-by-step approach based on creating a safe and trusting therapeutic relationship is crucial. Cognitive behavioral therapy (CBT) has proven to be particularly effective, especially techniques such as exposure therapy, cognitive restructuring, and social skills training. The goal of therapy is to change the negative beliefs and fear responses and promote safer, more realistic social interactions.

The inclusion of psychoeducational elements can also be useful in giving the patient a better understanding of the nature of the disorder and the coping strategies available. Group therapies can also be beneficial because they provide a safe environment where social skills can be practiced and positive social interactions can be experienced.

Asperger's syndrome (under autism spectrum disorder)

Asperger's syndrome is a neurobiological developmental disorder that is located within the autism spectrum. Those affected show significant abnormalities in social interaction and communication as well as stereotypical behaviors and interests. The syndrome was named after the Austrian pediatrician Hans Asperger, who first described it in 1944.

One of the central characteristics of Asperger's syndrome is the challenge in social interaction. Those affected often have difficulty understanding and using non-verbal communication such as facial expressions, gestures and eye contact. They also find it difficult to recognize social norms and subtle interpersonalities and to react adequately to them. This often leads to misunderstandings and difficulties in social interaction, which can affect the formation and maintenance of relationships.

The communication difficulties manifest themselves not only in non-verbal communication, but also in verbal communication. Individuals with Asperger's syndrome tend to take language literally. Metaphors, sarcasm and irony often cause them problems. Conversations are often perceived as one-sided, as those affected tend to talk about their specific interests and have difficulty taking into account the part of the conversation and the interest of the interlocutor.

Another characteristic feature of Asperger's syndrome is stereotypical and repetitive behaviors, as well as intense and specific interests. These areas of interest can be very complex and detailed, and sufferers often devote a significant amount of their time and attention to these issues. However, these intensive interests can also be used as a resource to support and promote learning and work processes.

Motor clumsiness or coordination difficulties are also more common in people with Asperger's syndrome. This can manifest itself in an unpolished gait, difficulties in learning fine motor skills or generally limited physical mobility.

Diagnostically, Asperger's syndrome today occurs within the umbrella term of autism spectrum disorders (ASD) according to the criteria of the DSM-5 (Diagnostic and Statistical Manual of Mental Disorders) and ICD-11 (International Classification of Diseases). That is, there is no longer a separate diagnosis of "Asperger's syndrome", but it is considered part of the spectrum of autism disorders.

Therapy for Asperger's syndrome is tailored to the specific needs of those affected and often includes behavioral and talk therapies, social skills training, and possibly pharmacological support. The aim is to improve social understanding and communication skills as well as to develop strategies for coping with everyday life. Any comorbid disorders such as anxiety disorders or depression are also addressed.

Attachment theory

Attachment theory, developed by John Bowlby in the 1950s, has profound implications for our understanding of how early relationships affect human development and behavior. Central to attachment theory is the assumption that people have the need from birth to form close emotional bonds with specific, usually primary caregivers, typically parents or guardians.

These bonds serve as a safe base for the child to explore their environment from, as well as a safe haven to return to in times of stress and threat. The quality of the bond between the child and its caregiver is significantly reflected in the way the child later enters into relationships with other people and responds to social, emotional and even cognitive challenges.

Mary Ainsworth expanded Bowlby's concept through her work in the 1970s, in particular through the development of the "stranger situation", an experimental paradigm for assessing the attachment security of young children. Her research identified various attachment patterns that were described as safe, insecure-avoidant, insecure-ambivalent, and later, through further research, disorganized attachment. A secure attachment pattern becomes recognizable when the child has confidence in the availability and sensitivity of the caregiver to his or her needs. Insecure attachment patterns often arise from inconsistent, unpredictable or negligent reactions of the caregivers to the needs of the child.

In the long term, the quality of early childhood bonds affects mental health, self-esteem, the ability to regulate emotions, and the stability of later attachment and love relationships. People with secure attachments tend to feel valuable and competent, have healthy stress management strategies, and effectively seek support and closeness in their relationships. People with insecure or disorganized attachments, on the other hand, may struggle to build trust, allow emotional intimacy, and develop effective strategies for managing stress.

In therapeutic practice, attachment theory is often used to understand the origin and patterns of a client's relationships. It provides insights into past attachment dynamics that can lead to current challenges and behaviors. This allows therapists to work specifically to identify and change these patterns in order to promote the client's emotional well-being and relationship skills.

Attention deficit/hyperactivity disorder (ADHD)

Attention deficit hyperactivity disorder (ADHD) is a neurobiological developmental disorder that typically begins in childhood and often persists into adulthood. It is characterized by persistent patterns of inattention, hyperactivity, and impulsivity that go beyond the developmental age of the sufferer.

Inattention

People with ADHD often show the following symptoms of inattention:

- Difficulty concentrating on tasks or games for long periods of time
- Common careless mistakes in schoolwork or other activities
- Problems organizing tasks and activities
- Avoidance or aversion to activities that require sustained mental effort
- Loss of items necessary for tasks or activities, such as toys, homework, pencils, books, or tools

- Easily distracted by external stimuli
- Forgetfulness in everyday life

Hyperactivity

Hyperactivity in ADHD often manifests itself through:

- Fidgeting or sliding around on the seat
- Leaving the seat in situations where sitting is expected
- Running around or climbing in inappropriate situations
- Difficulty playing quietly or keeping yourself quietly occupied
- Excessive talking
- Constant restlessness

Impulsiveness

Impulsivity is often manifested by:

- Blurting out answers before questions are fully asked
- Difficulty waiting for your turn in conversations or games
- Interrupting and disrupting others, such as when interfering in conversations or games

Causes and diagnosis

The exact causes of ADHD are not fully understood, but a combination of genetic, neurobiological, and environmental factors is assumed. Diagnosis is based on a thorough clinical evaluation, including a detailed medical history and observation of the person's behavior. Questionnaires and checklists, such as those included in the DSM-5 or ICD-10, are often used to assess the criteria.

Treatment

ADHD is usually treated through a combination of behavioral therapy, psychoeducation, and, in many cases, medication. Behavioral therapy approaches focus on strategies to improve self-regulation, organizational skills, and social skills. Psychoeducation helps those affected and their families to understand the disorder and deal with the challenges. Medications such as stimulants (e.g., methylphenidate) and non-stimulants can be effective in relieving the symptoms of ADHD.

Autism spectrum disorder

Autism spectrum disorder (ASD) is a neurobiological developmental disorder characterized by a variety of symptoms and characteristics. The term "spectrum" makes it clear that there is a wide range of symptoms and severity, so no two people with ASD are identical.

People with ASD often have difficulties in social interaction and communication. These difficulties can manifest themselves in a reduced ability to understand social cues, such as facial expressions, gestures or tone of voice. They often have trouble starting or maintaining conversations and may avoid non-verbal forms of communication, such as eye contact.

In addition, people with ASD often exhibit repetitive or restrictive behavior. This can manifest itself in the form of highly ritualized actions, limited interests, or obsessive preoccupations with specific issues. For example, they might spend hours studying model trains or have unusually detailed knowledge in a specific field.

Sensory hypersensitivities or undersensitivities are also present in many sufferers. This means that everyday sensory stimuli, such as light, sounds, touch or smells, can be perceived as overwhelming or unpleasant or, in contrast, hardly noticed.

The diagnosis of ASD is based on observation of behavior and an analysis of the affected person's developmental history. Professionals typically use standardized diagnostic tools such as the Autism Diagnostic Observation Schedule (ADOS) and the Autism Diagnostic Interview-Revised (ADI-R) to make an accurate diagnosis.

The causes of ASD are complex and multifactorial. It is assumed that genetic and environmental factors interact. Research shows that certain genetic mutations, as well as prenatal and perinatal factors, can increase the risk.

There is no cure for ASD, but various therapeutic approaches and support measures can significantly improve the quality of life. Behavioral and speech therapies, social skills training, and specialized educational programs are often helpful. Interdisciplinary care that covers all areas of life can also be of great benefit.

Adapting the environment can also have significant positive effects. Individually tailored strategies to manage sensory hypersensitivity, creating structured and predictable daily routines, and adapting learning or workplace environments are examples of this.

Societal acceptance and understanding of ASD has increased in recent decades, which has led to better support structures and more inclusive approaches to education and work.

Autogenic training

Autogenic training is a relaxation method developed by the Berlin psychiatrist Johannes Heinrich Schultz in the 1920s, which is based on the principles of self-hypnosis. This technique aims to achieve a profound relaxation of the body and mind through targeted focus on physical sensations and suggestive formulas. This is done primarily through the training of one's own perception and the ability to self-regulate.

The method consists of six standard exercises, which in turn are based on three basic building blocks: the gravity exercise, the heat exercise and the breathing exercise. Other exercises focus on the heart, abdomen and head. All exercises are designed to promote soothing deep relaxation and at the same time positively influence the vegetative functions of the body.

1. **Gravity exercise**: Here, the practitioner focuses his attention on the thought "My right arm is very heavy" (can vary, e.g. left arm or both legs). This concentration promotes muscular relaxation, which ultimately leads to a feeling of heaviness in the aforementioned parts of the body.
2. **Heat exercise**: This includes suggestions such as "My right arm is all warm." The aim is to increase vasodilation and blood circulation through this

mental focus, which leads to a subjective sensation of warmth.
3. **Breathing exercise**: In this exercise, the focus is on the breath and the suggestion "My breath flows calmly and evenly". This is intended to calm down the breathing process, which has an overall relaxing effect.
4. **Heart exercise**: The practitioners concentrate on their heart and formulas such as "My heart beats calmly and evenly". The aim is to calm the cardiovascular system.
5. **Solar plexus exercise**: This exercise focuses on the solar plexus with formulas such as "My solar plexus is pouring warm". This exercise aims to relax the internal organs and calm the digestive system.
6. **Head exercise**: Here, a cool forehead is suggested with formulas such as "My forehead is pleasantly cool", with the aim of bringing about mental freshness through this mental suggestion.

Autogenic training can be learned in both individual and group settings. A trained trainer or therapist initially guides clients through the exercises and supports them with verbal guidance and support. With time and regular practice, individual participants can apply the techniques independently.

The regularity of the exercise is an essential factor for the success of the training. Short, daily exercise sessions of about 5-15 minutes can already promote a significant improvement in well-being and stress management. Autogenic training is often used to treat stress, psychosomatic complaints, sleep disorders, mild to moderate anxiety disorders and depressive moods.

On a deeper level, it can also contribute to self-reflection and self-knowledge. The participants not only learn how to put themselves in a more relaxed state, but also how to feel themselves better and deal more consciously with their body sensations and emotional states.

Automatisms

The term "automatisms" refers to a series of unconscious, routine and usually stereotypical behaviors, thought processes or emotional reactions that take place without conscious control. These automatisms can have both adaptive and maladaptive functions.

In their adaptive form, automatisms make everyday life easier by saving energy and cognitive resources. An everyday example of this would be driving a car: After a certain amount of practice, humans learn and automate many of the necessary sequences of actions, so that complex processes can be carried out without conscious attention.

Maladaptive automatisms, on the other hand, are behavioral or thought patterns that can lead to problems in the long term. A classic example of this is compulsive actions or thoughts in obsessive-compulsive disorder. These are recurring, mostly senseless activities or beliefs that cannot be stopped voluntarily despite the knowledge of their absurdity or harmfulness.

Automatisms play an important role in many therapeutic approaches. In behavioral therapy, they are often identified as dysfunctional behavioral patterns and modified through targeted interventions, such as exposure or cognitive restructuring. In psychoanalytic or depth psychology-based therapy, the origin of these automatisms is often sought in unconscious conflicts or early childhood experiences and brought into consciousness through therapeutic work.

Another example of automatisms can be found in schema therapy, where certain automatic reaction patterns are described as schema modes. These modes can include emotional, cognitive, and behavioral automatisms and can be triggered by specific triggers that go back to previous maladaptive experiences.

Automatisms are also important in mindfulness practice. Here, an attempt is made to raise awareness of automated reactions by practicing mindfulness of one's own thoughts, feelings and actions. Through this increased awareness, automatisms can be recognized and replaced by conscious, reflected decision-making processes.

Insights into automatisms come from various fields of science, including psychology, neurobiology, and cognitive science. Neuroscientific research shows that automatisms are often caused by repeated activations of certain neuronal networks in the brain, making these networks work more efficiently and less resource-intensively.

The understanding and therapeutic processing of automatisms are therefore central to psychotherapy, as they are often the threshold beyond which short-term coping leads to long-term change and improvement in psychological well-being.

Avoidance behavior

Avoidance behavior is a psychological phenomenon in which individuals develop active or passive strategies to avoid unpleasant or fearful situations, thoughts, or feelings. These behaviors can take a variety of forms, including physical avoidance of places or people, cognitive repression of distressing thoughts, or the use of substances to numb unpleasant emotions.

In therapy, avoidance behavior is often understood as a maladaptive coping strategy. People often tend to use avoidance behaviors as a short-term solution to stress or anxiety because it provides immediate relief. In the long term, however, it contributes to the maintenance and possibly intensification of psychological problems because the underlying fears and conflicts are not dealt with, but merely circumvented.

A classic example of avoidance behavior is agoraphobia, in which sufferers avoid public places or crowds of people because they are afraid of panic attacks. Another example is social phobia, where socially anxious individuals avoid social interactions to prevent embarrassing or unpleasant situations.

The maintenance of avoidance behaviors is often promoted by negative reinforcement. This means that the sense of relief that comes from avoiding an anxiety-inducing situation reinforces the behavior itself, making it more likely that it will continue to be used in the future. This short-term relief reinforces the cycle of avoidance and prevents the confrontation and resolution of deeper psychological conflicts.

Therapeutically, the aim is usually to reduce avoidance behavior and replace it with more adaptive coping strategies. Cognitive behavioral therapy (CBT) and exposure therapy are commonly used methods to break the vicious cycle of avoidance. In exposure therapy, the affected person is systematically and controllably confronted with the fear-triggering stimuli in order to gradually reduce the fear reaction and strengthen confidence in their own coping abilities.

An important aspect in the treatment of avoidance behavior is also the reflection and awareness of one's own inner experiences. By fostering mindfulness and emotional awareness, the sufferer can learn to accept and tolerate their emotions instead of avoiding them. This contributes to the development of a more resilient, less fear-driven way of life.

Behavioral therapy

Behavioral therapy is a basic psychotherapeutic direction that focuses on the systematic change of dysfunctional behavior and thought patterns. It is based on learning theory principles and aims to achieve concrete and measurable changes in the experience and behavior of patients. This form of therapy assumes that problematic behavior is learned and can therefore be "unlearned" or replaced by functional behaviors.

A central component of behavioral therapy is behavioral analysis, which closely examines the patient's problematic behavior and the conditions that maintain it. Special attention is paid to triggering and maintaining factors. The therapist uses this information to develop individual therapy goals and tailor-made intervention strategies.

Behavioral therapy techniques include social skills training, in which patients learn to improve their communicative skills and find their way to assertive behavior. Exposure and confrontation therapy is also an important method, for example in the treatment of anxiety disorders, in which patients are gradually confronted with the anxiety-triggering stimuli in order to achieve habituation and reduction of anxiety.

Another central element of behavioral therapy is cognitive techniques that focus on identifying and restructuring dysfunctional thoughts and beliefs. This is about recognizing illogical and negative thought patterns and replacing them with more realistic and positive thoughts. This is often done through techniques such as cognitive restructuring, in which the patient learns to critically question their automatic thoughts and consider alternative interpretations.

Behavioral therapy is strongly empirically oriented and attaches great importance to the scientific verification of its methods and techniques. Through continuous research, their effectiveness and the effectiveness of individual interventions are constantly being optimized. Studies show that behavioral therapy can be successfully used to treat a variety of mental disorders, such as depression, anxiety disorders, eating disorders, and obsessive-compulsive disorder.

The therapist-patient relationship in behavioral therapy is cooperative and transparent. The collaboration is based on a clear structure and a goal-oriented approach, with the therapist providing the patient with specific tools and strategies so that they can actively participate in their change process. The patient is thus not regarded as a passive recipient of therapy, but as an active participant who contributes significantly to his or her own therapeutic success.

In behavioral therapy, homework is often used, in which patients practice new behaviors or ways of thinking outside of therapy hours and integrate them into their everyday lives. This practice of self-help promotes personal responsibility and sustainability of the therapy results.

Behaviorism

Behaviorism is an influential school of psychology that focuses in particular on observable behavior and its modification by environmental influences. This branch of psychology refuses to deal with internal mental states or processes that cannot be directly observed and measured. Instead, behaviorism emphasizes that all behaviors are learned and acquired through interactions with the environment.

The founder of behaviorism is John B. Watson, who formulated the basic principles of this theory in the early 1910s. Watson argued that psychology as a scientific discipline could only produce valid findings if it focused on objectively measurable and observable phenomena. Watson's work was later further developed by B.F. Skinner, who introduced the concept of operant conditioning.

Behaviorism distinguishes between different forms of learning, including classical conditioning and operant conditioning. Classical conditioning, studied in detail by Ivan Pavlov, describes the process by which a neutral stimulus triggers a conditioned response through repeated association with an unconditioned stimulus. An example of this would be Pavlov's famous experiment in which dogs began to salivate at the sound of a bell if food was previously regularly presented following the sound of the bell.

In operant conditioning, the modification of behavior through consequences is in the foreground. B.F. Skinner showed through his experiments that behavior can be shaped by reinforcement (reward) or punishment. Behaviour that has positive consequences tends to be shown more often, while behaviour that has negative consequences occurs less frequently. Skinner developed different reinforcement plans to explore the effects of different reinforcement types and intervals on behavior.

Essential to behaviorism is the idea that behavioral change can be achieved through targeted manipulation of environmental conditions. Therapeutic approaches that emerged from behaviorism use techniques such as systematic desensitization, flooding, and aversion therapy to reduce or eliminate unwanted behavior and promote desired behavior.

Systematic desensitization, for example, focuses on the step-by-step confrontation with anxiety-inducing stimuli, combined with the practice of relaxation techniques in order to gradually achieve desensitization to these stimuli. Flooding, on the other hand, confronts the patient suddenly and intensively with the anxiety-inducing stimuli until the fear reaction subsides.

Although behaviorism has been criticized, especially for its ignorance of internal mental processes and its mechanistic view of the human being, it has had a lasting influence on psychotherapy. Many of its principles have been integrated into modern cognitive behavioral therapies that take into account both environmental influences and cognitive processes.

Behaviorism thus remains a fundamental and historically significant paradigm in psychology and psychotherapy, which has paved the way for numerous other developments and therapeutic techniques.

Behavioural change

Behavior change refers to the process by which a person modifies their behavior to act more functionally or to achieve specific goals. This process can take place both consciously and unconsciously and is often the central goal of many psychotherapeutic approaches. Behavior change usually occurs through different stages of motivation, planning, action, and maintenance.

In psychotherapy, behavioral changes can be promoted through various therapeutic methods and techniques. These include behavioral therapy, which aims to identify dysfunctional behaviors and replace them with constructive behaviors. For example, in the case of a patient suffering from anxiety disorders, the therapist may use techniques such as exposure training. Here, the patient is exposed to the anxiety-triggering situations in a targeted and step-by-step manner in order to reduce the fear reaction and learn new, adaptive behavior patterns.

Another important component of behavior change is strengthening self-regulation skills. This includes strategies for self-monitoring and self-evaluation, such as keeping diaries or using reward systems to reinforce positive behaviors. Learning and practicing coping strategies that help the patient deal with stress and setbacks also plays an essential role here.

The process of behavior change is often complex and not linear, as relapses are common. However, a relapse is not seen as a failure, but as part of the change process, which provides important insights into the underlying difficulties and obstacles. Therefore, psychotherapeutic work places particular emphasis on promoting resilience and developing sustainable coping strategies.

Motivational interviewing can also be used to strengthen the patient's intrinsic motivation to change behavior. This approach emphasizes collaboration and supports the patient in exploring ambivalences about behavior change and formulating their own arguments for change. A key concept here is building self-efficacy, the patient's belief that they have the ability to successfully change their behavior.

In addition, cognitive behavioral therapy techniques, such as identifying and changing dysfunctional thought patterns, can serve as a support for behavior change. By learning to question and modify their thoughts and beliefs, patients can develop a more positive mindset that makes it easier to implement and maintain new behaviors.

Binding Types

In psychotherapy, attachment types play a crucial role in understanding the emotional and interpersonal behavior of patients. Attachment theory, originally developed by John Bowlby and later refined by Mary Ainsworth and other researchers, describes how the quality of early childhood attachment to primary caregivers influences later social and emotional behavior. There are four main categories of attachment types: safe, insecure-avoidant, insecure-ambivalent, and disorganized.

Secure Binding Type

Children with a secure attachment type usually have reliable and consistent emotional support from their caregivers. These children feel safe when their caregivers are around and can use them as a safe base to explore the world. Adults with secure attachment often have positive views of relationships and can tolerate both closeness and independence well. They tend to have healthy, balanced relationships.

Insecure-avoidant attachment type

Children with an insecure-avoidant attachment type often show a clear avoidance behavior towards their caregivers. These children have learned to suppress their emotional needs, as their caregivers may have been emotionally dismissive or fickle. They often seem self-reliant and independent, but avoid deep emotional ties. In adulthood, this behavior can manifest itself as emotional distancing and difficulties in managing relationships.

Insecure-ambivalent attachment type

Children with an insecure-ambivalent attachment type experience their caregivers as unpredictable in their emotional availability. They often react with high levels of fear and insecurity when separated from their caregivers, and exhibit behaviors that fluctuate between clinging and rejecting. Adults with this attachment type can have intense and often demanding relationships. They tend to be dependent and insecure in their relationships and are often afraid of being abandoned.

Disorganized attachment type

The disorganized attachment type often occurs in children who have experienced traumatic experiences or abuse at the hands of their caregivers. These children exhibit confusing behavior, characterized by fear and contradictory actions. They don't know how to feel safe, and their caregivers are a source of comfort and fear at the same time. In adulthood, individuals with this attachment type can have extreme difficulties in interpersonal relationships, often characterized by high levels of anxiety and lack of emotional coordination.

Knowing the different types of attachment allows psychotherapists to better understand the dynamics in their patients' relationships and to develop individual therapeutic approaches that correspond to the specific needs and difficulties created by the respective attachment experiences.

Binge Eating Disorder

Binge eating disorder (BED) is a clinically significant eating disorder characterized by repeated episodes of uncontrollable, disproportionately rapid, and massive consumption of large amounts of food in short periods of time. These binge eating attacks typically occur at least once a week over a period of at least three months and are associated with considerable suffering and loss of control. Those affected often experience strong feelings of shame and guilt after the binge eating, which further increases the stigma and emotional suffering.

In contrast to bulimia nervosa, binge eating disorder is not accompanied by compensatory behaviors such as vomiting, excessive exercise or the abuse of laxatives. This difference is of central diagnostic importance, as permanent overeating often leads to significant health problems such as obesity, type 2 diabetes, high blood pressure and cardiovascular disease.

Psychodynamically, BED is often understood as a coping mechanism that serves to temporarily regulate complex and unpleasant emotions such as grief, anger, loneliness or chronic stress. However, this mechanism leads to a vicious circle, as short-term emotional relief is bought by long-term psychological and physical damage.

Behavioral aspects of the disorder include unhealthy eating habits, ritualized behaviors, and eating in isolation. Those affected often report a "trance state" during their binge eating, in which they feel they cannot control consumption. In order to calm down after such episodes, emotional and cognitive stress can subsequently increase, which increases the risk of renewed binge eating.

The treatment of binge eating disorder requires a multidisciplinary approach that includes both psychotherapeutic and medical components. Cognitive behavioral therapy (CBT) is one of the most effective therapies for treating BED. CBT works to identify and modify dysfunctional thought patterns and behaviors to promote healthier eating behaviors and improve emotional management of stress. Other therapeutic approaches may include dialectical behavioral therapy (DBT), interpersonal therapy (IPT), and mindfulness-based techniques.

Drug therapy can also play a role, especially if there are concomitant mental illnesses such as depression or anxiety disorders. Antidepressants, such as selective serotonin reuptake inhibitors (SSRIs) and certain appetite suppressants, can help regulate eating behavior and stabilize mental health.

Comprehensive treatment often includes nutritional counseling and the development of an individualized eating plan to promote healthy eating habits and help people achieve a good balance with food. Physical activity is considered a complementary component of therapy, which can improve physical health and reduce psychological stress.

Patient care must be provided in an environment that provides support and understanding to reduce shame and guilt. Support groups and support networks can be a valuable resource that reduces feelings of isolation and provides community coping strategies.

Biofeedback

Biofeedback is a method in psychotherapy and health promotion that aims to give people the ability to perceive and consciously modify unconscious physiological processes. These procedures are based on the monitoring and feedback of physiological functions such as heart rate, muscle tension, skin conductance, respiratory rate and brain activity.

The central mechanism of biofeedback is that patients are connected via sensors to specific devices that measure physiological signals in real time and provide visual, auditory or tactile feedback. Through this feedback, often in the form of graphics or sounds, patients receive immediate feedback about their current physiological state and the changes they can bring about through various mental or physical exercises.

In therapeutic sessions, biofeedback is often used to help patients alleviate or control certain ailments, such as chronic pain, migraines, anxiety, high blood pressure, and stress. By learning how to change their physiological responses through techniques such as relaxation, breathing, and imagination, patients gain greater control over their physical and emotional states.

A typical biofeedback scenario could involve a patient with chronic headaches. The therapist places electrodes on the patient's scalp that measure muscle tension. The patient sees on a monitor how the muscle tension increases or decreases. Through targeted relaxation exercises, under the guidance of the therapist, the patient can immediately observe how the muscle tension and thus his headache is reduced.

Biofeedback can also be useful in treating anxiety. For example, heart rate variability feedback can help the patient identify when they are entering a state of heightened arousal and regulate that state by applying relaxation techniques or breathing exercises.

Through continuous practice and the use of biofeedback, patients can learn to use these techniques independently and more efficiently, which can lead to long-term improvement in health. The practice is often supplemented by behavioral therapy or cognitive interventions to ensure more comprehensive therapy.

Bipolar disorder

Bipolar disorder, also known as manic-depressive disorder, is a severe and complex mental illness characterized by extreme fluctuations in mood, energy, and activity. These fluctuations are far more intense and longer-lasting than the normal mood swings that most people experience.

A hallmark of bipolar disorder are the so-called manic and depressive episodes. During a manic episode, sufferers experience a greatly increased mood and excessive energy drive. This phase can be characterized by increased self-confidence, reduced need for sleep, increased urge to talk and an increased willingness to take risks. Sometimes this leads to impulsive and ill-considered actions that can have negative consequences.

In contrast, a depressive episode is characterized by the deepest depression, loss of interest, listlessness and hopelessness. Those affected are often unable to cope with everyday tasks and withdraw socially. In severe cases, suicidal thoughts can occur.

Bipolar disorder can occur in different forms:

1. **Bipolar I disorder**: In this case, sufferers experience at least one manic episode, which is often severe enough to require hospital treatment. Depressive episodes are not necessary for diagnosis, but they do occur frequently.
2. **Bipolar II disorder**: This form is characterized by the occurrence of at least one hypomanic episode and one major depressive episode. Hypomania is a milder form of mania that does not require hospital treatment, but still goes well beyond normal mood levels.
3. **Cyclothymic disorder**: It involves chronic fluctuations between hypomanic and depressive symptoms that are not intense or long enough to be classified as manic or depressive episodes. However, these fluctuations must last for at least two years.

The exact cause of bipolar disorder is not yet fully understood, but it is believed that a combination of genetic, biological, and environmental factors play a role. Neurotransmitter imbalances, structural and functional abnormalities in the brain, and familial clusters indicate a genetic predisposition.

The diagnosis of bipolar disorder is made through a thorough clinical evaluation, in which the psychotherapist determines a detailed life and medical history of the patient. Sometimes, questionnaires and scales are also used to determine the type and severity of symptoms.

Treatment for bipolar disorder aims to stabilize the mood swings and prevent future episodes. This is usually achieved through a combination of medication and psychotherapy.

Medications such as mood stabilizers, anticonvulsants, and antipsychotics are often the basis of pharmacological treatment. In addition, psychotherapies such as cognitive behavioral therapy (CBT), interpersonal therapy (IPT) and psychoeducational therapy are used to improve coping strategies and prevent relapses.

An important aspect of therapy is also the promotion of a regular rhythm of life and the avoidance of triggering factors such as lack of sleep and stress.

Bipolar Rapid Cycling

Bipolar rapid cycling is a specific form of bipolar disorder in which the sufferer experiences four or more episodes of mania, hypomania, mixed states, and/or depression within a year. This rapid succession of mood swings poses a significant challenge for both the affected person and treating therapists.

In mania, the patient experiences elation, increased energy, a desire to talk, and a reduced need for sleep, often associated with excessive self-confidence and impulsive actions. Hypomania is a milder form of mania in which the symptoms are less severe and there is less interference with everyday functioning.

In contrast, patients suffer from sadness, lack of energy, sleep disorders, low self-esteem and, in severe cases, suicidal thoughts during depressive episodes. Mixed states are particularly complex because they have characteristics of both mania and depression at the same time. Patients can suffer from extreme agitation and depressed mood at the same time, which often leads to considerable suffering.

The causes of bipolar rapid cycling are multifactorial and can include genetic predispositions, neurological changes, and environmental factors. It is suspected that dysregulation in the neurotransmitter systems, especially with regard to dopamine and serotonin, plays a role. Hormonal fluctuations, especially thyroid dysfunction, and psychological stressors could also influence the occurrence of rapid cycling.

For diagnosis and treatment, a careful patient history is crucial to capture the frequency and intensity of episodes. Treatment can be pharmacological and therapeutic. Lithium remains a drug of choice, supplemented by antidepressants and antipsychotics. Regular blood level monitoring may be necessary to monitor the effects and side effects of the medication. Psychotherapeutic approaches, such as cognitive behavioral therapy (CBT), social rhythm therapy, and psychoeducation, aim to promote stable life patterns, develop stress management strategies, and support medication adherence.

The prognosis and course of bipolar rapid cycling can vary. Some patients experience a decrease in episode frequency over time, while others experience a persistent, oscillating pattern. Switching between episodes can be unpredictable and abrupt, making it difficult to plan and execute effective therapeutic interventions and requiring a high degree of flexibility and adaptability from therapists.

Borderline Personality Disorder

Borderline personality disorder (BPD) is a complex mental illness characterized by a persistent pattern of instability in interpersonal relationships, self-image, and affects, accompanied by a marked impulsivity. People with BPD experience profound emotional fluctuations that are often perceived as overwhelming and difficult to control.

One of the central characteristics of borderline is the fear of abandonment. Those affected can make extreme efforts to avoid actual or perceived abandonment. This fear can lead to intense and often inappropriate reactions, such as excessive anger or panic at real or perceived rejections.

In interpersonal relationships, borderline can lead to a pattern of unstable and intense relationship experiences. Individuals with BPD tend to either idealize or devalue others, which often changes abruptly. This tendency towards the "black and white" perception of people, also known as splitting, can put a considerable strain on relationships and lead to repeated crises.

The self-image of people with borderline is often unstable and incoherent. They often struggle with an uncertain or distorted self-concept, which leads to difficulties in forming their identity. This insecurity can manifest itself in abrupt changes in professional goals, values, and sexual orientation.

Impulsivity is another central characteristic of borderline. Sufferers may exhibit high-risk behaviors such as uncontrolled spending of money, sexual risky behavior, substance abuse, reckless driving, or binge eating. These behaviors can serve as coping strategies in the short term, but lead to significant problems in the long term.

Emotional dysregulation is also a hallmark of BPD. Those affected experience intense and disproportionate emotional reactions to everyday events. They can manifest themselves in inappropriate anger, intense sadness, or overwhelming fear. These emotional fluctuations are often difficult to predict and can last from a few hours to a few days.

A tendency to self-injurious behavior, such as cutting, burning or even suicide attempts, is not uncommon in people with borderline. Such actions are often used as a means to cope with intense emotional pain or to combat an inner state of emptiness and meaninglessness.

Separation of reality and changes in perception are also possible. In extreme stressful situations, sufferers may experience paranoid ideas or dissociative symptoms, such as the feeling of unreality of the self or the environment.

Treatment for borderline personality disorder often focuses on a combination of psychotherapy and drug intervention. Dialectical Behavioral Therapy (DBT) and Mentalization-Based Therapy (MBT) are among the specialized therapeutic approaches that aim to promote emotional stability, improve relationship patterns, and increase impulse control.

A close, trusting therapeutic relationship is important because it serves as a safe framework within which patients can explore and change their relationship dynamics and emotional responses. Working with people suffering from BPD requires patience, empathy and a high willingness to self-reflect from therapists.

Bowlby, John

John Bowlby was a British psychiatrist and psychoanalyst whose work contributed significantly to the development of attachment theory. His research and theories have had a profound impact on psychotherapy, especially in the fields of developmental and clinical psychology.

Bowlby viewed attachment as a biologically anchored behavioral system that increases an infant's chances of survival by ensuring closeness to a caregiver. This attachment behavior manifests itself in signals such as crying, smiling and following, which serve to ensure the attention and closeness of a caring person. The relationship that develops between a child and its primary caregiver – often the mother – forms the basis for the emotional and social growth of the individual.

According to Bowlby's theory, children develop different attachment styles based on their early relationship experiences. These attachment styles can be divided into four categories: secure attachment, insecure-avoidant attachment, insecure-ambivalent attachment, and disorganized attachment. Securely attached children show confidence and seek security and comfort from their caregivers. Insecure-avoidant children tend to suppress their feelings and distance themselves from the caregivers. Insecure-ambivalent children exhibit contradictory behaviors characterized by insecurity and fear. Disorganized children exhibit a mix of behaviors that do not reveal a consistent style, often due to traumatic experiences or erratic care situations.

Bowlby postulated that these early attachment experiences have a significant impact on a person's emotional and mental health in adulthood. Extrapolations of his theory show that people with a secure attachment tend to have healthier and more stable relationships in their childhood than adults. In contrast, insecure or disorganized attachment experiences can lead to difficulties in emotional regulation, relationship problems, and increased risk of mental disorders such as depression and anxiety disorders.

His work also led to the realization that psychotherapeutic interventions may be necessary to treat the traumas and attachment injuries that arose in childhood. Bowlby-inspired attachment-oriented therapies aim to promote secure attachments and identify and reorganize existing insecure attachment patterns. This is often done by working on the therapeutic relationship between client and therapist, which can serve as a corrective emotional experience.

Bowlby was convinced that attachment was a lifelong process. Attachment patterns developed in childhood can be altered through significant new relationships and therapeutic interventions in adulthood. His research and theories have not only revolutionized psychotherapy, but have also had far-reaching implications for the understanding of interpersonal relationships in the broader social context. Attachment theory today serves as a fundamental concept that shapes our understanding of the role of early experiences and their influence on our mental health.

Brain function

Brain function refers to the complex and diverse processes that take place within the brain to control behavior, thinking, emotions, and physical responses. These processes include a variety of specific functions that are served by different brain regions and neural networks.

On the one hand, the prefrontal cortex plays a central role in the executive function. It is responsible for higher cognitive processes such as decision-making, problem-solving, planning, and the regulation of impulses. Through complex neural circuits, the prefrontal cortex orchestrates the ability to pursue long-term goals and resist short-term rewards.

Furthermore, the limbic system, which includes structures such as the hippocampus and the amygdala, is crucial for emotions and memory. The amygdala plays a key role in the processing and expression of emotions such as fear and anger, while the hippocampus is instrumental in the consolidation of memories and spatial memory.

The basal ganglia, another critical neural network, affect movements and motor control. They work together with the cerebellum, which is also involved in fine-tuning and coordinating movements. This interaction enables fluid and targeted movements.

Another important area is the occipital lobe, which is primarily responsible for vision. Here, visual stimuli from the eye are processed, interpreted and integrated with other sensory information. At the same time, the temporal lobe plays a major role in the processing of auditory information and language, especially through the Wernicke's area, which is central to language comprehension.

The parietal lobe, on the other hand, processes sensory information from different parts of the body and integrates it into a coherent spatial awareness. This fusion of information makes it possible to understand the position of one's own body in space and the relationship to objects and other people.

The brainstem structures, consisting of the midbrain, bridge and medulla oblongata, control essential life-supporting functions such as breathing, heartbeat and reflexes. The brainstem also serves as a communication hub between the brain and spinal cord, which allows for smooth transmission of sensory and motor signals.

Bridge of Affect

The affect bridge is a concept from depth psychological and psychoanalytic psychotherapy that serves to understand and use the connection between current emotional reactions and previous experiences or childhood experiences. The term is derived from the Latin "affectus", which means "feeling" or "emotion", and "bridge", a transition or connecting element.

In therapeutic practice, the therapist uses the affect bridge to be able to lead the patient from feelings and affects experienced in the present to previous experiences and memories that are emotionally and psychologically similar. This is often done through targeted questions or by focusing on specific emotions that occur during the session. If the patient experiences a strong feeling, such as fear, anger or sadness, the therapist will address this feeling and thus draw on previous experiences in which similar emotions have occurred.

The affect bridge method is based on the assumption that present emotional reactions do not exist in isolation, but often reflect experiences deeply rooted in the past. For example, a patient who is afraid in a current situation could be led through the affect bridge to a childhood experience in which he felt similar fear, possibly in interaction with an authoritarian parental figure. By reliving and becoming aware of such previous experiences within the safe framework of the therapeutic relationship, the patient can develop a better understanding of their current emotional reactions.

Another important aspect of the affect bridge is its ability to make unconscious or repressed memories more accessible. Often these memories are not immediately present in the patient's consciousness, but can be brought to light "like a bridge" by evoking and experiencing strong affects. Immersion in these memories enables the patient to recognize and work through unconscious conflicts that influence his or her current behavior and experience.

During this therapeutic process, it is crucial that the patient recognizes and understands the connection between current feelings and past experiences. This allows him to see the emotional intensity of current situations in a new light and to break through possibly dysfunctional patterns. The therapist works in a supportive and guiding manner to ensure that the patient is able to make and process these often difficult connections.

Bulimia Nervosa

Bulimia nervosa, a serious eating disorder, is characterized by repeated episodes of binge eating and subsequent compensatory behaviors such as vomiting, excessive use of laxatives, fasting, or excessive physical exercise. These behaviors typically occur at least once a week over a three-month period.

During an episode, a person may consume an exceptionally large amount of food in a relatively short period of time and feel that they have lost control of food. The amount of food consumed is significantly higher than what most people would consume under similar circumstances.

The compensatory behavior results from intense fear of gaining weight and from a distorted self-image, in which body weight and body shape excessively influence self-esteem. This behavior is intended to prevent the food eaten from having a negative effect on body weight.

The psychological side effects of bulimia nervosa often include shame, guilt and deep dissatisfaction with one's own body. Those affected often suffer from depression, anxiety disorders and low self-esteem.

Physiologically, the repeated binge eating and the subsequent compensatory behavior can have serious health effects. Common consequences are electrolyte imbalances, which can lead to cardiac arrhythmias and kidney problems. Tooth damage due to regular vomiting, inflammation and tears of the esophagus as well as chronic gastrointestinal problems are also common.

The diagnosis of bulimia nervosa is based on the criteria of the DSM-5 (Diagnostic and Statistical Manual of Mental Disorders, 5th edition) and requires a careful medical history and, if necessary, a physical examination, as well as laboratory tests to evaluate the health consequences.

Treatment usually involves a combination of psychotherapy, nutritional counseling, and sometimes drug therapy. Cognitive behavioral therapy (CBT) is one of the most commonly used forms of therapy and aims to change dysfunctional thoughts and behaviors. The therapy process promotes the development of healthier eating habits and a more realistic perception of body weight and body shape.

Long-term success in the treatment of bulimia nervosa often requires comprehensive support, including follow-up care and involvement of the social environment. A multidisciplinary approach that takes into account medical, psychological and nutritional aspects is essential for a sustainable recovery.

Burnout syndrome

Burnout syndrome describes a state of emotional, physical, and mental exhaustion that is often caused by chronic stress and overload at work. This condition is characterized not only by persistent fatigue and reduced performance, but also by increasing depersonalization and emotional numbness to one's own work and environment.

The development of burnout syndrome is often insidious and is usually divided into three phases. In the first phase, those affected experience a strong enthusiasm and a high willingness to perform, which, however, can quickly turn into excessive demands. This overload leads to the second phase, which is characterized by fatigue, irritability and reduced self-esteem. In the third phase, deep exhaustion takes place, accompanied by physical and psychological complaints such as headaches, sleep disorders, depressive moods and emotional exhaustion.

The causes of burnout syndrome are manifold and can lie both in the working conditions and in the personal disposition of the person affected. Factors such as a high workload, lack of recognition, lack of control over one's own work and a lack of a social support network play a central role. On an individual level, perfectionism, overcommitment, lack of boundaries and lack of stress management strategies can significantly increase the risk of burnout.

Burnout syndrome is diagnosed on the basis of a detailed medical history in which both professional and personal stress factors are considered. Questionnaires and clinical interviews are often used to obtain a comprehensive picture of the symptoms and their effects on everyday life.

The therapeutic treatment of burnout syndrome aims to provide both short-term relief and recovery and to bring about long-term changes that prevent a recurrence. The focus is on the development and implementation of strategies for stress management and the promotion of a healthy lifestyle. Various therapeutic approaches can be used here, such as cognitive behavioral therapy, mindfulness-based techniques and relaxation techniques. In severe cases, drug treatment may also be considered, especially if depressive symptoms are present.

Preventive measures also play an important role in dealing with burnout. This includes promoting a healthy working environment, building and maintaining social networks, and training managers in recognizing and addressing stress symptoms in employees at an early stage. Individually, prevention means above all recognizing and respecting personal boundaries, incorporating regular recovery phases and developing healthy coping strategies.

Cash register office

A health insurance registered office refers to the authorization of a psychotherapist in private practice to offer and bill services within the framework of statutory health insurance (GKV). This authorization requires the approval of an Association of Statutory Health Insurance Physicians (KV), which decides on the allocation of health insurance seats according to strict criteria. Owning a health insurance company is an essential prerequisite for many psychotherapists to be able to run their practice economically, as it ensures a stable patient base and a reliable source of income.

A health insurance company is closely linked to the admission to statutory health care. Psychotherapists who have this license undertake to treat a certain number of patients who have statutory health insurance. The billing of the services provided is carried out directly by the Association of Statutory Health Insurance Physicians, which calculates the fees on the basis of a fixed point system. This ensures that psychotherapeutic services are nationwide and accessible to all insured persons.

The path to a health insurance company can be lengthy and demanding. Usually, a university degree in psychology or medicine as well as a recognized psychotherapeutic training are required. After that, the license to practice psychotherapy must be obtained. The application for a health insurance seat can then be submitted to the responsible Association of Statutory Health Insurance Physicians. Often there are more applicants than available seats, which is why many psychotherapists have to wait years for a license.

An alternative to obtaining a new cash register is to take over an existing cash register from a colleague who is retiring. This often happens as part of a practice takeover or partnership. Various factors such as the location of the practice, the number of patients and the profitability of the practice play a role in this. The takeover must also be approved by the Association of Statutory Health Insurance Physicians.

A cash register office also includes the obligation to comply with certain obligations and regulations. This includes participation in statutory health care, regular training and compliance with quality standards. In addition, psychotherapists must periodically participate in quality controls and audits to ensure continuous quality assurance of the services offered.

The health insurance seat is not only a formal authorization, but also symbolizes a responsibility towards patients and the health care system. It ensures that patients have access to qualified psychotherapeutic treatment and that therapists can pursue their professional activities under fair and regulated conditions.

In conclusion, it can be said that the registered office plays a central role in the professional life of a psychotherapist, as it forms the basis for the treatment of patients with statutory health insurance and thus represents an essential basis for the operation of a practice.

Catharsis

Catharsis is a central term in psychotherapy, which comes from ancient Greek and originally meant "purification" or "purification of the soul". In therapeutic contexts, catharsis describes the process by which a person experiences liberation and relief through the expression and reliving of emotions, especially repressed or repressed feelings.

The cathartic process often takes place on a deep emotional level and can be triggered by various therapeutic techniques, including psychoanalysis, Gestalt therapy, depth psychology or humanistic therapeutic approaches. These techniques help the individual to bring buried emotions or painful memories to light and process them in a safe and supportive environment.

An essential part of catharsis is the conscious experience and expression of emotions such as sadness, anger, fear or pain, which have often been suppressed or ignored for a long time. Through this process, the physical and psychological tensions that arise from the suppression of these emotions can be released. People often experience significant relief and clarity after a cathartic session, which can lead to improved emotional and mental health.

However, catharsis is not always a goal in itself and should not be misunderstood as a quick or easy way to heal. Rather, it is a complex and sometimes painful process that should be carried out under expert guidance and in a safe, supportive environment. The primary purpose of catharsis is to restore emotional balance and help the individual to gain a deeper understanding of himself and his emotional world.

From a therapeutic point of view, catharsis can also play an important role in uncovering and processing trauma. Many trauma therapies, such as EMDR (Eye Movement Desensitization and Reprocessing) or somatic experience, include elements of emotional release. By processing and acting out the suppressed traumatic experiences, those affected can experience long-term healing and integration.

Child and Adolescent Therapy

Child and adolescent therapy refers to a specified area of psychotherapy that focuses on the treatment of emotional and psychological problems in children and adolescents. This form of therapy takes into account the unique developmental needs, cognitive abilities and emotional life situations of the young patients.

In the context of child and adolescent therapy, a variety of therapeutic approaches are used to treat various mental disorders. These can include bipolar disorder, anxiety disorders, depression, behavioral disorders, attention deficit/hyperactivity disorder (ADHD), and autism spectrum disorders. The therapeutic approach can include cognitive behavioral therapy, play therapy methods, systemic therapy, family therapy, and other techniques.

An essential component of child and adolescent therapy is the involvement of the family environment. Parents and other close caregivers often take an active role in the therapeutic process, as the family context can have a significant influence on the psychological state of the child. Family therapies and family training can be used to improve family dynamics and create supportive environmental structures for the child.

An age-appropriate and individualised approach is essential in the work with children and young people. Younger children often benefit from playful interventions through which they can express their emotions and feelings. Therapeutic games, drawings, puppetry, and other creative expressions are common tools that are used. For adolescents, on the other hand, it may make more sense to rely more on verbal and cognitive techniques in order to better understand and cope with their problems.

Another important aspect of child and youth therapy is the close cooperation with institutions such as schools, kindergartens or youth welfare offices. This cooperation ensures holistic support for the child by ensuring that all relevant actors act in sync.

In addition, child and adolescent therapy aims to strengthen emotional resilience and coping strategies in the long term. It does this by promoting self-esteem, social skills, and emotional intelligence. The treatment is designed to not only provide short-term relief from symptoms to the young patients, but also to develop skills that will help them in life permanently.

The diagnostic phase in child and adolescent therapy is particularly intensive and often includes a variety of diagnostic tools to identify the specific challenges and strengths of the child. Diagnostic interviews, observations, questionnaires and standardised tests are used to obtain a comprehensive picture of the psychological situation.

Preventive approaches also play a role in child and adolescent therapy. Early intervention is intended to identify and treat potential mental health problems before they develop into serious disorders.

Chronobiology

Chronobiology is a scientific discipline that deals with the temporal organization of biological processes and phenomena in the body. These processes usually follow periodic, often cyclical patterns that take place in roughly 24-hour rhythms, also known as circadian rhythms. These internal timers control a variety of bodily functions such as sleep-wake cycles, hormone secretion, body temperature, and metabolic processes.

A central component of chronobiology is the study of the so-called "internal clock," which is mainly located in the hypothalamus of the brain, more precisely in the suprachiasmatic nucleus (SCN). This internal clock synchronizes the internal biological processes with the external environmental conditions, such as light and temperature. Light, perceived through the eyes, serves as the main timer that adjusts the internal clock and influences the activity of the cells.

Chronobiology plays an important role in psychotherapy, especially when it comes to the treatment of sleep disorders, depressive episodes or seasonal affective disorders. In people with depression, for example, studies show that there is a shift in circadian rhythms. For example, the rhythm of the sleep hormone melatonin may be delayed, leading to sleep disorders and a deterioration in well-being. A therapeutic intervention that is often used is light therapy. Here, the patient is ideally exposed to intense artificial light in the morning to adjust the internal clock and stabilize his rhythms.

Another area of application of chronobiology in psychotherapy concerns so-called social jet lag. This refers to the discrepancy between an individual's biological clock and the socially required schedule, for example through working hours or social obligations. A chronobiological examination can help to analyze individual sleep patterns and develop strategies to improve well-being and performance.

Chronobiology also extends to long-term rhythms such as the circannual cycle, which includes annual cycles. Such rhythms could be influenced by seasonal changes in light and temperature, which can manifest itself, for example, in seasonal fluctuations in mood and behavior.

Clinical psychology

Clinical psychology is a branch of psychology that deals with the diagnosis and treatment of mental disorders, emotional problems, and behavioral problems. It combines theoretical and practical approaches to understand human behavior and to carry out individual and group-related therapeutic interventions.

At its core, clinical psychology deals with the study of mental disorders such as depression, anxiety disorders, schizophrenia, eating disorders and personality disorders. In addition, it includes the study of behavioral problems that affect interpersonal relationships, adjustment disorders and emotional stress.

An essential part of clinical psychology is diagnostics. Various methods such as clinical interviews, psychometric tests and behavioral observations are used to create a comprehensive picture of an individual's mental health. Diagnosis facilitates the development of an individual therapy plan tailored to the specific needs of the patient.

Different approaches and techniques are used in therapeutic practice. Among the best known are behavioral therapy, cognitive behavioral therapy, depth psychology, humanistic therapy, and systemic therapy. Each approach offers different tools and methods to treat mental disorders and improve patients' well-being.

Prevention also plays an important role. Clinical psychologists develop programs to prevent mental disorders and promote mental health through education and workshops. They often work together in multidisciplinary teams to offer holistic solutions to complex mental health problems.

Research is another central aspect of clinical psychology. It includes studies on the etiology (causal research), prevalence (frequency) and effectiveness of therapeutic approaches. This enables continuous improvement of therapeutic methods and a better understanding of mental illnesses.

Professionally, clinical psychologists work in a variety of settings, including hospitals, health centers, community-based facilities, psychiatric hospitals, schools, and private practices. They often work on an interdisciplinary basis with doctors, social workers, occupational therapists and other professionals to create holistic treatment plans.

The importance of clinical psychology in healthcare should not be underestimated. It makes a significant contribution to improving the quality of life and general well-being of people suffering from mental disorders.

Cognition

Cognition refers to the mental processes involved in receiving, processing, storing, and applying information. These processes include a variety of functions such as perception, attention, memory, thinking, problem-solving, decision-making, and language processing. In psychotherapy, understanding cognitions is central because they can greatly influence an individual's behavior and emotional states.

Perception is the process by which sensory information is transformed into a meaningful experience of the environment. It plays an essential role in that it is the first step in the process of absorbing information. Attention allows the individual to identify and focus on important environmental stimuli, filtering out irrelevant information. Memory is used to store information and experiences that can later be retrieved for orientation and decision-making.

Thinking involves manipulating information for problem-solving and decision-making. This can include both logical and creative thinking. Problem-solving is the application of knowledge and thought patterns to find a solution to a given challenge. Decision-making involves evaluating information and options to make a choice that appears to be the most effective or desirable.

An essential model for understanding cognitions in psychotherapy is the cognitive model according to Aaron T. Beck. It describes how negative thought patterns and beliefs, called cognitive schemata, can lead to emotional and behavioral problems. These negative patterns often influence automatic thought processes and can lead to a distorted perception of reality. By identifying and modifying these dysfunctional thoughts, therapists can support their patients to improve their emotional health and positively change their behaviors.

Another important concept in the field of cognition is metacognition, the examination of one's own thought processes. Metacognitive strategies help an individual monitor, control, and regulate their own cognitive activities to develop more effective problem-solving and learning methods.

Cognitive Behavioral Therapy (CBT)

Cognitive behavioral therapy (CBT) is a psychotherapeutic form of treatment based on the realization that our thoughts, feelings and behaviors are closely linked. It was originally developed by Aaron T. Beck in the 1960s and has continued to evolve since then. CBT is successfully used to treat a variety of mental disorders, including depression, anxiety disorders, eating disorders, obsessive-compulsive disorder, and post-traumatic stress disorder.

The central concept of CBT states that dysfunctional or distorted thought patterns can lead to emotional and behavioral problems. An important part of therapy is to identify these negative thought patterns, question them and replace them with more realistic and helpful thoughts. This process is called cognitive restructuring. The teaching of self-help techniques is also a central part of CBT, whereby the clients learn to change their thought patterns and behaviors in the long term and to improve them sustainably.

Another essential aspect of CBT is behavioral analysis, which examines specific behaviors and their motivational backgrounds. Through this analysis, problematic behavior patterns can be identified and replaced by targeted training of new, functional behaviors. The techniques include exposure exercises, in which clients are confronted with fearful situations in a step-by-step and controlled manner in order to achieve habituation or cognitive reassessment through learning psychology.

The therapeutic relationship also plays an important role in CBT, although it is primarily understood as a functional means of implementing the interventions rather than being the focus of the therapeutic process. The therapist does not act as an omniscient expert, but as a coach or companion who encourages the client to develop his or her own solutions and approaches.

A typical CBT meeting usually begins with setting an agenda and reviewing the homework done since the last meeting. This structured approach makes it possible to continuously evaluate progress and make adjustments if necessary. This is often followed by the processing of specific topics, using cognitive and behavioral therapy techniques.

The effectiveness of CBT has been well proven by numerous scientific studies. It is considered one of the most effective, evidence-based forms of therapy in many areas of mental health care. Another advantage of CBT is its comparatively short duration and its high structure, which makes it very easy to use, especially in outpatient care.

Cognitive dissonance

Cognitive dissonance describes the state of inner conflict that arises when a person has two or more conflicting beliefs, values, or insights at the same time. This condition leads to psychological discomfort, which motivates the person to reduce dissonance and restore cognitive harmony. The concept was developed in the 1950s by the social psychologist Leon Festinger and is one of the basic concepts of social psychology.

In detail, cognitive dissonance occurs when there is a discrepancy between a behavior and a belief, or between two beliefs. For example, a person who sees themselves as environmentally conscious may experience cognitive dissonance when flying, causing high CO_2 emissions. This discrepancy leads to an unpleasant tension.

There are several ways people can try to reduce cognitive dissonance:

1. Change of attitude:

A person might change their attitude so that it is more in line with their behavior. For example, it could adjust its stance on environmental compensation by convincing itself that flying is essential in certain situations.

2. Behavioural change:

The affected person could also change their behavior to align it with their beliefs. This could mean that she decides to fly less in the future or chooses alternative modes of transport.

3. Adding new cognitions:

Another strategy is to add new relevant cognitions that justify the existing behavior. For example, a person might take the position that they are offsetting flight behavior through other environmentally friendly actions, such as driving an electric car or participating in reforestation projects.

4. Minimizing Meaning:

Finally, the person may reduce the importance of dissonant cognition. She could tell herself that her individual contribution to climate change is small and therefore not so significant.

Recognizing and understanding cognitive dissonance is of great importance in psychotherapy because it provides insights into the way clients deal with inner conflict and how they may maintain maladaptive behaviors or thought patterns. Therapists can use this mechanism in a targeted manner to support clients in identifying and changing dissonant thought patterns, which is an important step towards a more inclusive and coherent self-perception.

For example, clients might find themselves in problematic relationship patterns perpetuated by cognitive dissonance by maintaining a certain image of themselves or their partner despite seeing opposing evidence. Through interventions that include both cognitive and behavioral elements, therapy can help uncover and re-evaluate dissonant cognitions, which can lead to significant improvements in well-being.

Cognitive restructuring

Cognitive restructuring is a therapeutic technique that is mainly used in the context of cognitive behavioral therapy (CBT). Their primary goal is to identify, question, and replace dysfunctional or irrational thought patterns with helpful and more realistic thoughts. This process aims to mitigate emotional and behavioral problems that result from negative thought patterns.

The cognitive restructuring approach is based on the assumption that thoughts, feelings, and behaviors are closely linked. Dysfunctional mindsets, such as exaggerated generalizations, black-and-white thinking, or catastrophizing thoughts, can lead to emotional distress and problematic behaviors. When these negative thoughts are persistent and recurrent, they can lead to chronic emotional problems such as depression, anxiety disorders, or obsessive-compulsive disorder.

To begin cognitive restructuring, the therapist first helps the client identify their negative automatic thoughts. This requires mindfulness and introspection, often aided by techniques such as keeping a thought log. A thought log is a tool in which the client notes down situations that trigger unpleasant emotions, accompanied by the corresponding automatic thoughts and the resulting feelings.

Once these thoughts have been identified, they are systematically questioned and checked for their reality content. This is done through techniques such as Socratic conversation, in which the therapist guides the client through targeted questions to examine the rationality and justifiability of his thoughts. Other techniques include gathering evidence to the contrary to refute the negative thoughts, or developing alternative, more positive beliefs.

The final stage of cognitive restructuring is to integrate the knowledge gained into everyday life. The client learns to apply and consolidate the new, more functional ways of thinking in real situations. This can be done through role-playing, homework, or practicing new thought patterns.

Coma

A coma is a state of deep unconsciousness in which a person cannot be woken up by external stimuli, nor does he show spontaneous movements or purposeful behaviors. This condition can be caused by a variety of causes, including severe head injuries, strokes, poisoning, infections, or metabolic disorders. In psychotherapy, coma is primarily considered in the context of the effects on the mental health and rehabilitation of the affected person.

A coma is classically defined in stages that reflect the depth and nature of the impairment of consciousness. This classification can be done according to the Glasgow Coma Scale (GCS), which assesses the patient's motor responses, verbal responses, and eye openings. A low GCS value indicates a deeper coma.

While the patient is in a coma, the therapeutic team works in an interdisciplinary manner to ensure the best possible care and prognosis. These include measures for pressure relief, infection control and nutrition, as well as physiotherapy interventions to prevent muscle atrophy and contractures.

Psychotherapeutic work after waking up from a coma requires a deep understanding of the neuropsychological consequences and the potential changes in the personality and cognitive abilities of the affected person. Often, the post-coma phase requires intensive rehabilitation that focuses on restoring basic functions such as language, motor skills, and memory. Psychosocial aspects such as reintegration into the family and the social environment also play an important role.

The psychotherapeutic support of relatives is another central part of the work with a patient in a coma. Relatives often experience intense emotional stress, which can range from hope and despair to fear and grief. Therapeutic support and counselling can help to get through these difficult times and improve the quality of life of the entire family.

Longer-term psychological consequences after a coma can take various forms, such as post-traumatic stress disorder, depression or anxiety. The treatment of these conditions requires precise diagnostics and individually tailored treatment approaches, which can range from cognitive behavioral therapy to drug support and integrative approaches.

Completion of therapy

The conclusion of therapy refers to the formal and emotional conclusion of psychotherapeutic treatment. This process marks the end of the regular sessions and the patient's transition from intensive therapeutic cooperation to independent handling of the strategies and findings developed. The completion of psychotherapy represents a significant milestone for both the patient and the therapist.

The conclusion of therapy begins long before the actual last session. At this time, the therapist should systematically prepare the process of closing with the patient. This involves a joint reflection of the therapy goals that were defined at the beginning of the treatment. The therapist and patient work together to evaluate the progress and successes of the treatment, as well as the remaining challenges. Through this review, what has been achieved is highlighted and appreciated, which strengthens the patient's self-worth and confidence in his own abilities.

An important part of the completion of therapy is the stabilization of the therapeutic progress achieved. Here, the techniques and coping strategies learned during therapy are once again specifically consolidated. The patient is encouraged to use these techniques in future stressful situations as well. This can be done through role-plays, hypothetical scenarios, or discussing specific upcoming events.

The emotional aspect of the conclusion of therapy is just as important. The therapist should create space for processing the feelings related to the end of therapy. The conclusion can be accompanied by a mixture of joy about the progress made and sadness about the end of the therapeutic relationship. Openly addressing and validating these feelings supports the patient in the processing process.

In the course of completing therapy, a so-called relapse prevention plan is often also drawn up. This plan includes specific strategies and guidance on how the patient can deal with possible relapses or difficult times. This includes identifying warning signs that could occur in the run-up to a possible relapse. Together, therapist and patient develop concrete steps to take in such situations.

Finally, completing therapy also provides an opportunity to talk about the future and how to maintain progress in the long term. The patient is guided to maintain a sustainable lifestyle that supports their mental health. This includes encouragement to use social support systems, establish regular self-care practices, and take other supportive measures as appropriate.

A successful conclusion of therapy requires both good preparation and a sensitive and reflective approach. It allows the patient to leave the therapy with a sense of completeness and strengthened self-efficacy and strengthens the likelihood of long-term therapeutic success.

Conditioning

Conditioning is a central term in behavioral therapy and describes the process by which an individual learns a specific response to a specific stimulus. This learning process takes place through repeated experiences and can be divided into two main forms: classical conditioning and operant conditioning.

Classical conditioning, which goes back to the work of Ivan Pavlov, is the process in which a neutral stimulus (e.g. a sound) is presented in pairs with an unconditioned stimulus (e.g. food). After several pairings, the neutral stimulus alone begins to trigger a similar reaction (e.g. salivation) as the unconditional stimulus. The neutral stimulus thus becomes a conditional stimulus. A classic example of this is Pavlov's experiment with dogs, in which he showed that a bell sound that originally caused no response, after repeated coupling with the sight of food, eventually triggered the dogs' salivation.

Operant conditioning, which has been studied extensively by B.F. Skinner, describes the learning of behaviors through consequences. Here, a behavior is modified by reinforcement (or punishment). Positive reinforcement involves adding a pleasant consequence (for example, praise or a reward) to increase the likelihood that the behavior will be repeated. Negative reinforcement involves removing an unpleasant consequence (for example, stopping a loud noise) to reinforce a behavior. Punishment, on the other hand, aims to reduce undesirable behaviors through negative consequences.

The principles of conditioning have far-reaching applications in psychotherapy. They are often used to change problematic behavior patterns or to learn new, adaptive behaviors. In exposure therapy, for example, classical conditioning is used to reduce clients' anxiety responses to anxiety-inducing stimuli. This is achieved by repeated, controlled exposure of the affected person to the fear-inducing stimulus, in the absence of the feared consequences, which can lead to the deletion of the fear response.

Operant conditioning is also used in a therapeutic context, especially in behavioral modification techniques. Therapists often work with reinforcers such as praise, rewards, or token systems to encourage desired behaviors. Understanding a client's individual motivations and reinforcers is crucial for the success of the therapy.

Conditioning not only explains how behavioral patterns can be learned and changed, but also provides valuable insights into how human learning and behavior work. This makes them an essential concept in psychotherapy and psychology in general.

Confabulation

Confabulation is a complex phenomenon that occurs primarily in neuropsychological and clinical practice. It refers to the unconscious invention of false or distorted memories in order to fill gaps in memory. These memories generated are often very real for the person concerned, although they are objectively false or falsified. Confabulation differs from deliberate lying in that the person concerned has no intention of deception and is firmly convinced that his or her stories are truthful.

Confabulation often occurs as a symptom of certain neurological and psychiatric disorders. The phenomenon is particularly well-known in connection with Korsakoff syndrome, a memory disorder caused by chronic alcohol consumption. Confabulation can also be observed in other conditions such as Alzheimer's dementia, frontotemporal dementia and certain forms of amnesia.

A distinction is made between spontaneous and provoked confabulation. Spontaneous confabulations occur without external stimulation and are often detailed and vivid. They can be very confusing for the affected person and their social environment, as they occur unexpectedly and seemingly incoherently. Provoked confabulations, on the other hand, occur in response to specific questions, when the person tries to give logical and coherent answers, even if he or she lacks actual memories.

The exact neurobiological mechanisms behind confabulation are not yet fully understood. However, it is suspected that damage or dysfunction in certain brain regions, such as the frontal lobe and the limbic system, play an important role. These areas are vital for the processing and storage of memories, as well as for the ability to self-examine and correct narratives.

From a therapeutic point of view, dealing with confabulations is a great challenge. It is important to adopt a respectful and empathetic attitude so as not to jeopardize the patient's trust. Direct confrontation or questioning of the fabricated memories can lead to increased confusion and emotional distress. Instead, it is often more helpful to support the person concerned in arranging their stories narratively and offering them tools for better orientation in the present.

As treatment progresses, it may also be useful to develop strategies to strengthen memory and cognitive control. This can be done through special memory training or psychoeducational measures that educate the patient and his relatives about the nature and mechanisms of confabulation.

Conflict of interests

A "conflict of interests" refers to a situation in which different interests, needs or goals of the parties involved contradict each other. In a psychotherapeutic context, this term can be applied both to the client-therapist dynamic and to internal conflicts within the client himself.

In the therapist-client relationship, a conflict of interests can arise if the client's goals are not in line with the therapeutic goals. For example, a client might be interested in quick, symptomatic relief, while the therapist is looking for profound, long-term change. Such discrepancies can have a significant impact on the therapeutic process and require open communication and negotiation to reach an amicable solution.

On the intrapersonal level, a conflict of interests can occur when different parts or needs are in conflict with each other within the client. A typical example is the inner conflict between the desire for independence and the need for closeness and security. Such inner conflicts can lead to considerable emotional and cognitive stress and often represent a central focus in psychotherapeutic work.

The identification of a conflict of interests is an important step in the therapeutic process. This includes analysing the interests, needs and values involved in detail and understanding the context in which they occur. Through techniques such as empathetic listening, reflection and targeted questions, the therapist can help the client to better understand his inner and outer conflicts.

Another element of dealing with conflicts of interests in therapy is the development of strategies for conflict management. This may mean finding compromises, reprioritizing or exploring alternative paths that cater to different interests. In some cases, it may also be necessary to temporarily put certain interests or needs on the back burner in order to get closer to an overarching goal.

A conflict-free state is rarely the ultimate goal of therapy, as conflict and conflicting interests are integral and unavoidable parts of life. Rather, therapy aims to provide the client with the tools and insights they need to deal with such conflicts in a constructive and healthy way. The promotion of resilience also plays an essential role in order to enable the client to better cope with future conflicts.

Confrontation

Confrontation is a psychotherapeutic technique that aims to directly confront clients with specific behaviors, thought patterns, or emotions that they may not be aware of or avoid. This technique is often used to enable insight and change by bringing unpleasant or repressed aspects into consciousness. It is an integral part of various therapeutic approaches, such as cognitive behavioral therapy, Gestalt therapy, and psychodynamic therapy.

Basically, confrontation is used to encourage clients to deal with their inner conflicts and contradictions. In cognitive behavioral therapy, this could be done by directly questioning irrational thoughts. For example, a therapist might directly confront a client suffering from social anxiety with the illogic of their negative automatic thoughts. Such an approach challenges the client to rethink their beliefs and develop alternative, less fearful thoughts.

In Gestalt therapy, on the other hand, confrontation aims to connect clients with their present experiences and feelings. The therapist often uses techniques such as role-playing or working with the "empty chair" to confront clients with unprocessed emotions or unfinished situations from the past. This promotes awareness and processing of these emotions in the here and now.

Within psychodynamic therapy, confrontation is used to uncover unconscious conflicts and defense mechanisms. For example, the therapist could focus on unconscious motives or early childhood experiences that influence the client's current behavior. This type of confrontation helps the client identify connections between past experiences and present problems, which can lead to a deeper understanding and potentially a breakthrough in therapy.

It is of particular importance that the confrontation always takes place in a safe and supportive therapeutic setting. The therapist must ensure that the client is sufficiently prepared and uses the confrontation in a measured manner in order to avoid excessive demands or additional psychological stress. A keen sense of timing and a trusting therapeutic relationship are therefore essential. Confrontational techniques should always be accompanied by empathy, understanding and respect for the client's individual boundaries and needs.

Constriction of consciousness

Constriction of consciousness refers to a state in which a person's consciousness is restricted in its scope and perception. This means that the affected person only perceives and experiences a limited part of the normally existing mental and emotional range. This constriction can have various causes and often occurs in stressful or traumatic situations.

Often, narrowing of consciousness manifests itself in a strong focus on certain thoughts, feelings or experiences, while other aspects of the experience or the environment are faded out. This concentration can happen involuntarily or arbitrarily. In extreme cases, a person in a state of constriction of consciousness may be fixated on a specific action or event, which prevents them from perceiving and processing other relevant information.

A classic example of constriction of consciousness is tunnel vision, which often occurs in extremely stressful or dangerous situations. Here, perception is focused so strongly that only the immediate threat or the direct impulse to act is at the center of consciousness. Other details of the environment that could contribute to a more comprehensive understanding of the situation are no longer registered.

In psychotherapy, narrowing of consciousness is treated, among other things, in the context of its diverse manifestations. These manifestations include states of panic, certain depressive episodes, but also dissociative states in which the consciousness is limited to limited experiences or memories. A particularly striking example is flashbacks in post-traumatic stress disorder (PTSD), in which the affected person is completely immersed in the traumatic memory and the present reality is temporarily pushed out of consciousness.

The therapeutic work with people who suffer from constriction of consciousness aims to gradually expand consciousness again. This is done through techniques of mindfulness, cognitive restructuring, and the safe recognition and processing of the underlying stress- or trauma-induced experiences. A central approach is to support the affected person in gaining control over their attention and consciously directing it to different aspects of their experience and environment.

Conversational psychotherapy

Conversational psychotherapy, also known as client-centered or person-centered therapy, is a form of psychotherapeutic treatment developed by Carl Rogers in the 1940s. It is based on the belief that every person has the ability and potential to understand and solve their own problems if they can act in a supportive and empathetic therapeutic relationship.

At the core of conversational psychotherapy is the assumption that mental disorders and personal conflicts result from incongruities between the person's self-image and his or her actual experiences. These discrepancies can lead to internal tension and emotional difficulties. The therapeutic process aims to reduce these incongruities and achieve greater congruence between the self-concept and the experiences.

A central element of conversational psychotherapy is the unconditional positive appreciation of the client by the therapist. This means that the therapist accepts the client without prejudice, evaluation, or criticism. This attitude fosters a sense of security and trust that allows the client to speak openly about their thoughts and feelings.

Empathy is another fundamental principle. The therapist strives to fully understand the client's perspective and understand their feelings. This goes beyond simple empathy and involves a deep, empathetic understanding of the client's inner world. Through this empathetic attitude, the client feels understood and often experiences relief from emotional pain.

Another important aspect of conversational psychotherapy is the authenticity or congruence of the therapist. This means that the therapist is honest and authentic in their interaction with the client. He does not hide behind a professional façade, but shares his real reactions and feelings in a way that serves the therapeutic process. This authenticity fosters an atmosphere of trust and sincerity.

The therapeutic process in conversational psychotherapy is non-directive, which means that the therapist does not give the client specific instructions or suggest solutions. Instead, he supports the client in gaining his own insights and making independent decisions. The client is seen as the expert for their own experiences, while the therapist acts as a companion and supporter in this self-exploration process.

Conversational psychotherapy places great emphasis on the quality of the therapeutic relationship and believes that this relationship is the primary remedy. By experiencing an accepting, empathetic and authentic relationship, the client can find new ways to deal with themselves and their difficulties. The emphasis is on strengthening the client's self-esteem and promoting their self-acceptance.

This form of therapy can be used for a variety of mental and emotional difficulties, including depression, anxiety, relationship problems, and stress management. It can also be used as a supplement to other therapeutic approaches and offers valuable support in personal development and self-discovery.

Countertransference

Countertransference is a psychoanalytic concept that was originally developed in the classical psychoanalysis of Sigmund Freud. It describes the emotional, often unconscious reactions and attitudes that a therapist develops towards a patient. These reactions can be both positive and negative in nature and can be strongly influenced by the therapist's personal experiences, traits and unresolved inner conflicts.

Countertransference plays a crucial role in the therapeutic process, as it can interfere with therapy if left unchecked. For example, the therapist may not perceive certain feelings of the patients correctly or may not respond to them appropriately. He could also unconsciously encourage or inhibit certain behaviors, depending on how his own inner conflicts collide with the patient's issues.

An example of countertransference could be when a therapist who experienced neglect as a child develops particularly strong protective feelings towards a patient who reports similar neglect. These feelings could lead the therapist to act overly caring and thus lose therapeutic neutrality. Alternatively, a therapist who carries his own unresolved anger may react to a certain provocative attitude of a patient with disproportionate bitterness or impatience.

Therapists must constantly reflect and analyze their own countertransference. This is often done in the context of supervision and self-analysis to ensure that their reactions and actions remain meaningful and helpful in the therapeutic process. Awareness of these reactions allows the therapist to act more empathetically and objectively, while deepening the relationship with the patient.

An alert approach to countertransference can prove to be a valuable diagnostic tool. By recognizing and understanding their own emotional responses, therapists can gain deeper insights into patients' dynamics and intervene in a more targeted manner. It also allows them to recognize unconscious messages or repressed emotions of the patient that could be reflected in the transference.

Couples Therapy

Couples therapy, also known as marriage counseling or couples counseling, is a form of psychotherapy that focuses on improving relationship dynamics between romantic partners. This form of therapy is usually led by psychotherapists, psychologists or specially trained counsellors and aims to resolve conflicts, improve communication patterns and strengthen emotional intimacy.

Couples therapy often begins with an inventory phase, in which therapists detail the history of the relationship, the individual backgrounds of the partners, and the specific issues that led them to therapy. This initial evaluation phase is crucial to understanding the dynamics and specific challenges of the relationship.

A central element of couples therapy is the improvement of communication between the partners. Misunderstandings and unspoken expectations are often the main causes of conflicts in relationships. Therapists therefore work intensively to help partners develop effective communication strategies. This can include techniques such as active listening, expressing one's needs and feelings in a non-confrontational way, and learning conflict resolution strategies that are respectful and constructive.

Another essential goal of couples therapy is to improve the emotional connection and understanding between partners. Many couples lose the ability to connect emotionally and support each other over time. Through various therapeutic interventions, such as remembering positive experiences together, practicing appreciation and overcoming challenges together, couples can regain the emotional depth of their relationship.

The therapeutic approaches in couples therapy can vary depending on the therapy model. The best-known approaches include behavioral couples therapy, emotion-focused couples therapy, systemic therapy and cognitive couples therapy. Each of these approaches offers specific methods and techniques for changing dysfunctional behavior patterns and strengthening relationship quality.

Behavioral couples therapy focuses on changing harmful patterns of behavior and encouraging positive interactions. Emotion-focused couples therapy aims to deepen emotional bonds and understanding of underlying emotional needs. Systemic therapy considers the couple as part of a larger social system and examines the interaction with it. Cognitive couples therapy focuses on recognizing and changing harmful patterns of thought and perception that lead to relationship problems.

The effectiveness of couples therapy depends on both the expertise of the therapist and the willingness of the partners to actively work on themselves and the relationship. Many couples report significant improvements in relationship quality, deeper emotional understanding, and better conflict management skills after couples therapy.

Course of therapy

The course of therapy encompasses the entire sequence and dynamics that extends from the first session to the conclusion of the therapeutic intervention. It begins with the initial phase, in which the therapist and the client build a trusting relationship, exchange basic information and gain an initial understanding of the problem. During this phase, the anamnesis, diagnostic measures and the determination of therapy goals are carried out.

In the further course, the work phase usually follows, in which the actual therapeutic work takes place. This phase is characterized by a variety of interventions and techniques, which can vary depending on the theoretical orientation of the therapist and the specific problem of the client. Cognitive behavioral therapy, depth psychology-based methods or systemic approaches are just some of the possible therapeutic models that can be used.

During therapy, the therapist constantly reflects on the process, progress and difficulties that arise. It is continuously evaluated how the treatment is progressing and whether adjustments are necessary. The therapeutic relationship remains a central element and, depending on the therapy model, can serve as a catalyst for change processes.

The course of therapy can also be characterized by so-called crises or turning points, which often mark significant advances or important breakthroughs. These events can be triggered by intense emotional experiences, confrontational sessions, or new insights from the client.

Finally, the course of therapy is characterized by the termination phase. In this phase, progress and changes are recapitulated, relapse prevention strategies are developed and the client is prepared for the time after therapy. The process ends with the formal termination of the sessions, but leaves open the possibility for future refresher sessions if deemed necessary.

Covering up psychotherapy

Covering psychotherapy is a therapeutic approach that aims to alleviate the symptoms of a mental illness or emotional problem without explicitly exploring or working on the underlying causes. In contrast to revealing therapy methods, which aim to raise awareness of deeper, often unconscious conflicts, cover-up psychotherapy focuses on the direct alleviation of symptoms and the management of current problems.

An essential part of covering psychotherapy is the use of techniques and interventions that are directly aimed at improving the patient's current condition. This can include various methods, such as behavioral therapy, psychoeducational approaches, or supportive techniques. The therapist helps the patient develop strategies that allow them to better manage their symptoms and function more effectively in their everyday life.

In covering psychotherapy, the stabilization of the patient plays a central role. This includes strengthening existing resources and resilience as well as promoting self-efficacy. The therapist works to enable the patient to reduce their discomfort and improve their quality of life, without necessarily initiating deeper, often more complex and possibly lengthy therapeutic processes.

Cover-up psychotherapy is particularly useful in crisis situations, acute psychological stress or patients whose resources are not sufficiently available for an intensive examination of profound psychological conflicts. In such cases, covering therapy can help to provide quick and targeted relief and create a basis for further therapeutic measures.

This form of therapy can also be a valuable addition to other, more intensive therapy methods. It can be used as a preparatory or accompanying measure in combination with uncovering therapies to first stabilize the patient and then, in a safer and more stable state, to enable him to work on his problems more deeply.

Overall, the focus of covering psychotherapy is on the here and now, on the elimination of acute complaints and the promotion of short-term improvements in mental state. This can be of great importance, especially in a modern society, which is often concerned with quick results. An important goal is that the patient is able to find a better way of dealing with his current challenges and to increase his quality of life in the long term, even if the deeper causes of his problems remain untouched at first.

Crisis intervention

Crisis intervention is a psychotherapeutic approach that is used when a person is experiencing an acute mental health crisis. A crisis should not be confused with everyday stress or challenges. It is characterized by an overwhelming feeling of being overwhelmed, in which the person's usual coping mechanisms fail. This can be triggered by a wide variety of life events, such as the loss of a loved one, the loss of a job, diagnoses of serious illnesses or traumatic experiences.

A mental health crisis can be characterized by signs such as intense anxiety, confusion, helplessness, panic, sadness, and in some cases, self-injurious behavior or suicidal thoughts. During such crisis phases, there is a great risk for the affected person to fall into a state of disintegration of psychological stability, which requires immediate and effective interventions.

The main objective of crisis intervention is to quickly restore a state of security and stability. The process often begins with an immediate assessment of the situation to understand the extent of the crisis and the person's acute needs. The therapist usually provides emotional support at first to alleviate feelings of isolation and despair. Active listening and empathetic understanding are crucial here.

An important part of crisis intervention is relief, also known as "de-escalation". Techniques are used to reduce the emotional arousal and tension of the affected person. This can be done through calm and clear communication, breathing exercises or other anxiety-relieving techniques.

Another critical component is problem reflection. The therapist helps the affected person to understand the causes and course of the crisis. This involves identifying resources and previous successful coping strategies that the affected person may be able to use. Together, they are working to develop an immediate response plan that aims to take concrete steps to address the crisis.

If necessary, the therapist can also assist in arranging additional help, whether through referrals to specialized professionals, by contacting social networks or by referral to inpatient treatment.

The effectiveness of crisis intervention depends largely on the timely and appropriate response of the therapist. The therapeutic process usually ends with the planning of aftercare to ensure that the person continues to be supported and can develop long-term strategies for crisis management.

Cyclothymia

Cyclothymia refers to a chronic affective disorder characterized by numerous periods of hypomanic and subdepressive symptoms. These symptoms are less pronounced than in bipolar disorder and do not meet the full diagnostic criteria for hypomanic or depressive episodes.

Hypomanic phases in cyclothymia are characterized by increased mood, increased energy and activity, and a decreased need for sleep. Sufferers may feel euphoric, expansive, or irritable, and often show increased self-esteem, a desire to talk, and unusually high productivity. However, these conditions are less likely to lead to the social or occupational impairments that occur in manic episodes of bipolar disorder.

The subdepressive phases, on the other hand, are characterized by persistent mild depressive symptoms. Sufferers experience a depressed mood, lack of interest in activities, decreased energy, and difficulty concentrating. However, these phases are not as intense or long-lasting as in major depressive disorder.

An essential feature of cyclothymia is the chronicity of the symptoms. In order to make the diagnosis, hypomanic and subdepressive phases must alternate repeatedly over a period of at least two years (one year in adolescents) without symptom-related free intervals lasting longer than two months. Cyclothymia can be associated with functional impairment, although the effects are often more subtle, characterized by chronic internal stressors and interpersonal difficulties rather than severe symptom spikes.

Sufferers can suffer from an unstable mood and emotional dysregulation, which often leads to problems in interpersonal relationships and in the professional environment. This constantly changing emotional state can represent a high degree of frustration and stress for those affected and their environment.

Treatment for cyclothymia usually includes psychotherapy and psychosocial interventions. Cognitive behavioral therapy (CBT) can help identify and change dysfunctional thought patterns. Interpersonal therapy (IPT) and other psychotherapeutic approaches can help to cope with interpersonal problems and increase emotional stability. In some cases, drug therapy, such as mood stabilizers or antidepressants, may also be considered, especially if the symptoms are significantly debilitating.

Since cyclothymia is often associated with an increased risk of developing bipolar disorder, long-term and continuous care by a psychotherapist or psychiatrist is important in order to monitor the course of the disease and initiate appropriate therapeutic measures in a timely manner.

Day clinic

A day clinic is a specialized facility in the field of psychotherapy that offers patients intensive therapeutic treatment during the day without them having to spend the night in hospital. It represents an interface between outpatient and inpatient care.

In the day clinic, patients are usually treated for several hours on weekdays, although the duration of the stay can vary depending on individual therapy needs. This structure allows patients to be in their familiar environment in the evenings and on weekends, which can facilitate the transition to everyday life. The therapeutic offers in the day clinic are diverse and often include individual and group therapies, art and design therapies, music therapy, movement therapy and relaxation techniques. Psychoeducational offers and social therapeutic measures are also often part of the program.

A major advantage of the day clinic is the intensive care provided by an interdisciplinary team of doctors, psychologists, social workers, nurses and therapists from various disciplines. This team works closely together to ensure a holistic approach to treatment and to respond individually to the needs of each patient.

A stay in a day clinic usually takes place after a thorough diagnostic clarification and is suitable for patients whose mental illness requires more intensive treatment than in purely outpatient therapy, but does not require continuous inpatient care. Typical indications for treatment in the day clinic can be severe depression, anxiety disorders, eating disorders, personality disorders and psychosomatic illnesses.

Another central aspect of the day clinic is the promotion of self-help skills and the improvement of everyday coping. Patients are given the opportunity to learn new coping strategies and to apply and try them out directly in their everyday lives. On the one hand, this is intended to establish behavioural changes more sustainably and, on the other hand, to avoid relapses more sustainably.

Due to the close-knit care and the structured day program, a day clinic also offers the opportunity to recognize crises at an early stage and to intervene in a targeted manner. This helps to mitigate severe courses and improve the prognosis of the mental illness.

Depersonalization

Depersonalization is a psychological condition in which the affected person feels alienated from themselves, their body or their mental processes. She experiences a persistent or recurring perception as if she were an observer of her own thoughts, feelings, perceptions and actions, but she feels as if she is detached from herself and her surroundings. The condition can be accompanied by feelings that affect one's body or identity, that are unpleasant or unsettling.

Patients suffering from depersonalization often report feelings as if they are "standing next to themselves" or separated from the rest of the world by an invisible barrier. Their thoughts and actions may seem strange or machine-like to them. They often feel a distance from their own emotions or notice that their environment is perceived as unreal or strange. These perceptual disorders can be associated with severe stress, anxiety or trauma and often occur in episodes that can last minutes to hours, but in severe cases they can persist for months.

During an episode of depersonalization, the affected person may have difficulty recognizing their actions as self-initiated. It can give the impression that they are following external mechanisms. These experiences can cause deep uncertainty and fear, especially if they are experienced for the first time.

Suffering from persistent or recurrent depersonalization can lead to the diagnosis of depersonalization-derealization disorder (DDS) in clinical practice, especially if the symptoms cause significant suffering or impair functioning in social, occupational, or other important areas. Diagnosis is often made by means of clinical interviews and diagnostic questionnaires. Experienced therapists also check for possible comorbidities such as anxiety disorders, depression or post-traumatic stress disorder (PTSD).

Treatment methods include behavioral therapy approaches and psychodynamic forms of therapy to help those affected identify and work on the underlying causes and triggers of depersonalization. Various techniques such as mindfulness training, grounding exercises, or teaching coping strategies can also be used to help deal with acute episodes of depersonalization. In some cases, drug treatment may be considered, especially if the depersonalization is accompanied by other psychiatric disorders.

Depression

Depression is a profound mental disorder characterized by persistent sadness, loss of interest or enjoyment of activities that one used to enjoy, as well as a variety of other emotional and physical symptoms. It is one of the mood disorders and can severely affect a person's daily life and functioning.

A major characteristic of depression is persistent depression. This is defined not only by the feeling of sadness, but also by feelings of emptiness, hopelessness and worthlessness. Affected people often report that they cannot see a way out of this state and that positive things in their lives become less important.

Another central symptom is the loss of pleasure and interest, also known as anhedonia. This applies to activities that used to be enjoyable, such as hobbies, social interactions, or even everyday tasks. This indifferent attitude towards activities can lead to withdrawal from social life and increase feelings of isolation.

Physical symptoms include significant changes in sleep patterns, such as insomnia or hypersomnia. Sufferers may either have difficulty falling asleep and staying asleep, or they may sleep an unusually large amount without feeling rested. Changes in appetite and weight are also common, although these can include both an increase and a decrease.

Loss of energy and constant fatigue are also characteristic of depression. The simplest everyday life can seem overwhelming, and the energy required for basic tasks can seem enormous. This is often accompanied by reduced ability to concentrate and difficulty making decisions, which can affect professional and academic performance.

Thoughts of death or suicide are particularly worrying in the context of depression. These can range from vague considerations about death to concrete suicide plans. It is therefore crucial that people in this situation receive professional support without delay.

The causes of depression are multifactorial. Genetic predisposition, biochemical imbalances in the brain, psychological factors such as traumatic experiences or chronic stress, and social influences such as isolation or stressful living conditions all play a role. Neurotransmitters such as serotonin, norepinephrine, and dopamine are often involved and can be affected by antidepressant medications.

Therapeutically, there are various approaches to treating depression. Psychotherapeutic methods such as cognitive behavioral therapy (CBT) aim to recognize and change negative thought patterns. Interpersonal therapy (IPT) and mindfulness-based procedures are also used. In more severe cases, drug treatment may be necessary, usually in combination with psychotherapy. Exercise, nutrition and social support are complementary measures that can promote the healing process.

Depth Psychology

Depth psychology is an important approach in psychotherapy that focuses on the exploration and treatment of mental problems by raising awareness of unconscious processes. Originally founded by Sigmund Freud, depth psychology encompasses several theoretical directions and therapeutic techniques, all based on the basic idea that many of our emotional and psychological problems are based on unconscious conflicts, desires, and memories.

A central concept of depth psychology is the unconscious. This psychic realm contains thoughts, memories, and feelings that lie outside of our conscious experience. Although they are not directly accessible to us, these unconscious contents influence our behavior, emotions, and interpersonal relationships in profound ways. Depth psychological therapy aims to bring these unconscious contents into consciousness in order to enable understanding and healing.

Another important concept is the defense mechanism. This concept describes psychological strategies that the ego uses to protect itself from fearful and unpleasant thoughts and feelings. For example, repression, denial, and projection are among the most common defense mechanisms. A depth psychology-oriented therapist helps clients to recognize their defense mechanisms and to understand how they influence the current behavior.

The therapy method in depth psychology is often more lengthy and intensive than other forms of therapy, as it aims to solve deep-rooted problems. The therapeutic process uses techniques such as free association, dream interpretation, and the analysis of the transference-countertransference ratio. Free association encourages the client to express all thoughts and feelings without censorship in order to uncover hidden content. Dream interpretation analyzes dreams as an expression of unconscious desires and conflicts, and the transference-countertransference relationship examines the emotional relationship between therapist and client, which often reflects past relationship patterns.

An important aspect of depth psychology work is the structural theory of the psyche, which includes the ego (the conscious level), the id (drives and unconscious needs), and the superego (inner morality and social norms). These three instances are in a dynamic field of tension with each other, and conflicts between them can cause psychological suffering. The depth psychology-oriented therapist tries to understand and treat these inner-psychic conflicts and the resulting symptoms.

Derealization

Derealization refers to a psychological phenomenon in which those affected perceive their environment as unreal, alien or distant. This experience can occur with various mental illnesses, including anxiety and panic disorders, post-traumatic stress disorder (PTSD), depressive disorders, and dissociative disorders, especially depersonalization-derealization disorder.

Sufferers often describe derealization as a feeling as if they are seeing "through a veil" or "as if in a dream". Their environment appears to them changed, depersonalized or surreal. Objects can appear distorted, color-altered, or like backdrops. This experience is often accompanied by a considerable feeling of uncertainty and fear, as those affected lose control of their perception and question their reality.

The occurrence of derealization can be favored by various factors. Acute stressful situations, trauma, extreme fatigue or substance effects, such as those that can occur when consuming drugs or alcohol, play a role. A genetic predisposition and neurobiological abnormalities can also increase the likelihood of derealization occurring.

Therapeutically, derealization is treated through various approaches. Behavioral therapy methods work to reduce anxiety and improve the perception of current reality, while cognitive techniques, such as the targeted questioning and restructuring of distorted thought patterns, can be helpful. Body-oriented procedures, such as mindfulness exercises and physical activities, help those affected to reconnect more strongly with their current environment. Psychotropic drugs, especially antidepressants and empathetic support from the therapist, can be used in addition to reduce the intensity of the symptoms.

Diagnosis

Diagnosis is a component of psychotherapeutic practice. It refers to the complex process in which a psychotherapist tries to obtain as precise a picture as possible of a patient's condition and symptoms on the basis of systematic observations, detailed discussions and standardised diagnostic procedures.

During the diagnosis, the therapist uses various tools and techniques to comprehensively record both the objective findings and the patient's subjective experiences. These include anamnestic interviews, in which the patient's life history and current problems are discussed, as well as psychometric tests, which depict specific characteristics and symptoms through standardized questions and tasks. Questionnaires such as the Beck Depression Inventory (BDI) or the Minnesota Multiphasic Personality Inventory (MMPI) are often used here.

Another important element of diagnosis is clinical assessment, in which an experienced therapist brings in his observations and experiences to interpret the patient's behaviors, emotional states, and cognitive processes. Diagnostics may also include medical examinations, especially if physical causes of psychological symptoms need to be ruled out or confirmed, such as through a physical examination or laboratory tests.

Diagnosis is usually made according to the criteria of common classification systems such as the Diagnostic and Statistical Manual of Mental Disorders (DSM-5) of the American Psychiatric Association or the International Classification of Diseases (ICD-10) of the World Health Organization. These systems provide standardized criteria that facilitate accurate diagnosis and understanding of complex disease patterns, and enable consistent communication between professionals.

In addition, the diagnosis makes it possible to develop tailor-made and evidence-based therapy plans that are based on the individual needs and strengths of the patient. It forms the foundation for the selection of suitable therapeutic interventions and supports the process of goal setting and follow-up within the therapy.

An ethically responsible approach to the diagnosis requires treating the patient with respect and empathy, taking his or her perspective seriously and involving him or her in the diagnosis. Openness and transparency in dealing with diagnostic findings promote trust and the therapeutic alliance, which can have a positive effect on the success of therapy.

Diagnostics

Diagnostics in psychotherapy refers to the structured process of recording and evaluating mental disorders, behaviors and emotional states of a patient. This procedure is essential to make a precise and well-founded diagnosis and to derive the appropriate therapeutic intervention.

At the beginning of the diagnosis, there is a thorough anamnesis, in which the clinical history of the patient is recorded. This includes current symptoms as well as previous mental and physical illnesses, family and social backgrounds as well as traumatic experiences. Various techniques and instruments are used, such as structured interviews, questionnaires and standardised tests.

Another central element of diagnostics is the observation of patient behavior in the therapeutic setting. The psychotherapist pays attention to nonverbal signals, emotional reactions and behavioral patterns that can provide valuable clues to the underlying psychological problems.

Psychometric testing plays an important role in diagnostics. Scientifically validated tests and scales are used to measure specific mental functions and disorders. Examples of this are intelligence tests, neuropsychological tests, personality tests and specific disorder tests such as for depression or anxiety disorders.

Another component of the diagnosis is the differential diagnosis. The therapist must carefully analyze all results in order to distinguish similar or comorbid disorders from each other. This requires not only extensive expertise, but also a high level of sensitivity and experience. It is checked whether symptoms are due to other medical or psychological causes to avoid misdiagnosis.

As part of the diagnosis, the patient's resources and strengths are also identified. This includes individually available coping strategies, supportive social networks and existing resilience factors. These resources are used specifically in therapy to support the change process.

The entire diagnosis is summarized in a treatment plan, which forms the basis for the therapeutic measures. This plan is flexible and is continuously reviewed and adapted during the course of therapy in order to be able to react to changes in the patient's condition.

The quality of the diagnostics is crucial for the success of the therapy. Through careful and comprehensive diagnostics, the therapist can obtain a detailed picture of the patient's mental state and design the therapy in a targeted and individual manner. The continuous review and adaptation of the diagnostic process ensures that the therapeutic measures are always tailored to the current needs and developments of the patient.

Dialectical Behavioral Therapy (DBT)

Dialectical Behavioral Therapy (DBT) is a specialized form of cognitive behavioral therapy developed by psychologist Marsha M. Linehan in the late 1980s. Originally designed for the treatment of borderline personality disorder, DBT has now been shown to be effective for other mental disorders, such as eating disorders, depression and post-traumatic stress disorder.

A central element of DBT is the notion of "dialectics," which essentially means that two seemingly contradictory things can be true at the same time. In therapy, this becomes concrete through the balancing act between acceptance and change. You work on embracing difficulties and painful emotions while working in parallel to change patterns of behavior and thinking.

DBT consists of four main components:

1. **Mindfulness**: Mindfulness techniques are the foundation of DBT. The aim here is to teach clients methods on how to stay in the here and now, to deal intensively with their thoughts, feelings and sensory experiences and not to judge them.
2. **Stress tolerance**: This component aims to provide patients with skills to manage and survive stressful or painful situations without developing destructive behaviors such as self-harm or impulsive action.
3. **Emotion Regulation**: These skill sets help clients reduce the intensity and duration of emotional responses and find healthy ways to manage and process strong emotions.
4. **Interpersonal effectiveness**: This focuses on improving relationships by learning skills on how to

express your needs in relationships clearly and directly, while setting healthy boundaries.

DBT therapies usually involve individual therapy sessions, group training, and telephone coaching. The individual sessions focus on the patient's specific problems and the application of the techniques learned. In group training, the core skills are taught and practiced. Telephone coaching is available to support the client in times of crisis and to encourage the application of the skills in real-life situations.

An essential part of DBT is the validation of the patient's experiences and feelings, which means that the therapist actively acknowledges and respects the client's perspective, which strengthens trust and the therapeutic relationship.

DBT requires therapists to have specific training and a deep understanding of dialectical theories and techniques. It is a methodologically structured, but also flexible form of therapy that is continuously tailored to the needs and progress of the patient.

Disorientation

An orientation disorder refers to an impairment of a person's ability to orient themselves in time, space, to their own person or situationally. This impairment can have various manifestations and causes and often occurs in connection with mental, neurological or somatic illnesses.

Temporal orientation disorder: In this case, the affected person has difficulty correctly recording or reproducing current times, dates or periods. This can mean that she cannot give a precise date and time or has problems correctly classifying the chronological sequence of events.

Spatial orientation disorder: Those affected lose the ability to find their way around in their environment. This can occur in familiar environments as well as in new, unfamiliar environments. The person can no longer find their way home or has difficulty grasping the structure of a room or building and using it sensibly.

Orientation disorder towards oneself: In this case, the affected person is not able to correctly state or recognize essential information about himself. This includes, for example, your own name, age, date of birth, address or other personal data. This form of disorder can cause particularly profound identity problems.

Situational orientation disorder: This type of orientation disorder refers to the understanding and classification of the current situation and its context. Affected individuals have difficulty grasping the significance of events or understanding the social expectations and norms in a given situation.

Orientation disorders often occur in the context of delirium, dementia, severe depressive episodes, schizophrenia or after a traumatic brain injury. They can occur acutely or develop insidiously and vary in their severity and effects depending on the diagnosis of the cause.

In the diagnosis, a detailed medical history is often collected and neuropsychological test procedures are used to determine the type and extent of the orientation disorder. Examples of tests are the Mini-Mental Status Test (MMST) or the clock sign test.

Treatment depends heavily on the underlying cause. In some cases, drug therapies may be indicated, such as for dementia or depression. In other cases, psychotherapeutic interventions, cognitive training or environmental measures that affect the orientation and self-positioning of the affected person are useful.

Promoting routines, a clear structure of the daily routine and an environment that is as clear and understandable as possible can help to give those affected a feeling of security and control. The support of relatives and nursing staff also plays an important role in coping with orientation disorders.

Dissocial personality disorder

Dissocial personality disorder, also known as antisocial personality disorder, is a profound and persistent personality disorder characterized by a consistent pattern of disregard and violation of the rights of others. People with this disorder usually show an imperviousness to social norms and legal rules, as well as a lack of empathy and remorse for their actions.

Sufferers tend to engage in repetitive, illegal or unethical behavior, which is often self-centered, impulsive, and manipulative. For example, they may be more likely to lie, steal, cheat, or use violence to achieve their goals, regardless of the consequences for others.

These behavioral patterns usually begin in childhood or early adolescence and continue into adulthood. Early signs such as truancy, animal cruelty, vandalism or other forms of aggressive behaviour often become apparent. A central trait is the inability to establish or maintain stable and peaceful relationships with other people.

The causes of dissocial personality disorder are complex and multifactorial. Genetic influences, neurobiological factors, environmental influences and difficult childhood experiences, such as neglect or abuse, play a role in this. Together, these factors can influence the development of the basic behavioral and personality traits that lead to the disorder.

The disorder is diagnosed through a thorough psychiatric history and an analysis of behavior over a longer period of time. Important diagnostic criteria include repeated criminal behavior, persistent dishonesty, impulsivity, irritability and aggressiveness, ruthlessness towards one's own safety, and the inability to learn from past negative experiences or take responsibility for one's own behavior.

Treatments for dissocial personality disorder are challenging, as those affected often have no insight into their problematic behavior and may not recognize the need for therapy. Psychotherapeutic approaches, especially cognitive behavioral therapy, can help to change harmful behavior and develop alternative coping strategies. In some cases, drug treatment can also help reduce aggressive and impulsive behavior.

Social professions, legal contacts and the relatives of those affected are often also involved in order to jointly create a supportive environment and practical solutions to the challenges posed by dissocial personality disorder.

Dissociative disorder

A dissociative disorder is a complex mental illness characterized by a separation of thoughts, memories, feelings, actions, or one's sense of identity. This is a decoupling of experiences that are normally connected and integrated. This separation can significantly impair normal consciousness and mental function.

Dissociative disorders cover a spectrum of different phenomena and are usually divided into different categories:

1. **Dissociative amnesia**: This form is characterized by the inability to remember important autobiographical information that would normally be easy to recall. This amnesia is often associated with a traumatic or highly stressful event and can only refer to certain periods of time, events or even the entire past.
2. **Dissociative Identity Disorder (DID):** Formerly known as multiple personality disorder, DID is characterized by the presence of two or more different personality states or identities. These identities can have different names, ages, genders, languages, and personality traits. In addition, memory lapses can occur that go beyond ordinary forgetfulness, indicating changing control by the different identities.
3. **Depersonalization/derealization disorder**: In depersonalization disorder, those affected experience their own person as foreign or unreal, while in derealization disorder the environment is perceived as unreal or distant. These experiences can often be very distressing and lead to considerable impairments in everyday life.

4. **Dissociative disorder unspecified (DSNNB):** This category includes various dissociative phenomena that cannot be clearly classified into the above categories. These include, for example, trans- and possession-like states, which can be culturally specific.

The cause of dissociative disorders is often attributed to extreme traumatic experiences, especially in childhood. These include physical, sexual or emotional abuse, extreme neglect, experiencing a natural disaster or other existential threats. The dissociative mechanism originally served as a protective function to emotionally distance the individual from unbearable experiences.

The diagnosis of dissociative disorders is challenging and includes a thorough anamnestic survey, exploratory interviews and sometimes specialized questionnaires or diagnostic interviews. It must be ensured that the symptomatology is not explained by other mental or neurological illnesses, and substance use must also be ruled out as a cause.

Therapeutically, dissociative disorders are usually treated with a combination of psychotherapy and possibly drug support. The aim of psychotherapy is to integrate traumatic memories and dissociative symptoms and to improve self-awareness and control. A trauma-focused form of therapy such as EMDR (Eye Movement Desensitization and Reprocessing) is often used. The therapeutic process includes stabilization, trauma processing and finally integration and rehabilitation.

Understanding and treating dissociative disorders requires great sensitivity and extensive clinical experience, as they are often associated with a variety of accompanying symptoms and comorbidities, such as anxiety disorders, depression, somatoform disorders or personality disorders. The establishment of a trusting therapeutic relationship is of particular importance in order to create a safe space for the often complex and painful processes of coming to terms with the past.

Disturbance of memory

Memory impairment refers to an impairment in the ability to store, retain or retrieve information. These impairments can occur in different severity and types and affect different areas of memory. Memory disorders can affect both short-term memory and long-term memory and manifest themselves through different symptoms, such as forgetting simple information or remembering past events.

In a clinical context, a distinction is made between different types of memory disorders, including amnesia and confabulations. Amnesia is memory loss that either occurs suddenly, for example after trauma, or progresses gradually, as is the case with neurodegenerative diseases. A distinction is made between retrograde and anterograde amnesia. Retrograde amnesia refers to the loss of memories of events before the point of occurrence of the disorder, while anterograde amnesia refers to the inability to form new memories after the damaging event.

Confabulations are false memories or the free invention of experiences, which those affected often unconsciously present as actual memories. These often occur in connection with neurological diseases such as Korsakoff syndrome.

The causes of memory disorders are manifold. They can be caused by physical damage to the brain, including traumatic brain injury, stroke, or tumors. Degenerative diseases such as Alzheimer's disease and other forms of dementia also play a central role. Psychological stress, such as depression or post-traumatic stress disorder (PTSD), can also lead to memory disorders.

From a therapeutic point of view, different approaches can be considered depending on the cause. In the case of neurological memory disorders, the focus is often on rehabilitative methods that aim to stabilize and promote remaining memory performance. Cognitive training programs, memory exercises, and assistive technologies such as memory aids can be used. Psychotherapeutically, the focus is, among other things, on the processing of traumas that have led to memory problems, as well as on dealing with the everyday problems and fears caused by the disorders.

An interdisciplinary approach is important in both diagnostics and therapy. Neurologists, psychiatrists, psychotherapists and occupational therapists often work together to provide comprehensive support to those affected. Diagnostic procedures include neurological examinations, neuropsychological test procedures and imaging procedures such as magnetic resonance imaging (MRI) or computed tomography (CT).

Documentation obligation

The documentation obligation in psychotherapy refers to the legal and professional ethical obligation of psychotherapists to keep detailed and precise records of the course of therapy, the treatment methods used, diagnoses as well as relevant observations and interactions with patients. This obligation serves a variety of purposes, from ensuring continuous and consistent treatment to legal safeguarding and quality assurance.

Thorough documentation begins with the anamnesis and diagnosis. Here, the patient's complaints, medical history, biographical data and diagnostic considerations are recorded. This lays the foundation for the creation of an individually adapted therapy plan, which is also documented. The treatment contract between therapist and patient, the defined therapy goals and the planned interventions are an essential part of these records.

In the course of the therapy, all sessions are documented. This includes not only a bullet-point summary of the conversation and the essential contents, but also a detailed description of the therapeutic measures carried out, techniques and the respective reaction of the patient to them. Progress and setbacks, changed symptoms, therapy adjustments and special incidents must also be noted. These continuous notes allow for clear traceability of the entire therapy process.

Furthermore, administrative aspects are also subject to the documentation obligation. This includes, in particular, records of appointments, agreed therapy breaks or terminations, as well as billing data and reports to cost bearers or referring bodies, such as family doctors or specialists.

The documentation obligation also includes data protection. Sensitive data must be kept strictly confidential and secured and stored in accordance with applicable data protection laws and professional ethics guidelines. Electronic documentation requires additional security measures, such as encrypted data storage and access rights, to ensure the protection of patient data.

Complete and careful documentation is also of great importance in the legal context. In the event of disputes or if a review by supervisory authorities is pending, the therapy documentation is important evidence. You can provide proof that the psychotherapist has fulfilled all necessary professional duties of care and has carried out the therapy responsibly.

Ultimately, the documentation obligation serves quality assurance in psychotherapeutic practice. It enables continuous evaluation and optimization of therapeutic work. By regularly reflecting on the documented content, the therapist can check the effectiveness of the methods used and, if necessary, make adjustments to ensure the best possible treatment for the patient.

Dream interpretation

Dream interpretation is a central concept in psychotherapeutic practice, which has established itself above all in the psychoanalytic tradition. Developed and popularized by Sigmund Freud, dream interpretation is a method in which dreams are analyzed to reveal hidden desires, fears, and conflicts of the unconscious.

Freud described dreams as the "royal road" to the unconscious. In his theory, dreams are divided into two levels: the manifest dream content and the latent dream content. The manifest dream-content is that which the dreamer consciously remembers and narrates as a dream. It is often veiled and subject to symbolic changes. The latent dream content, on the other hand, consists of the hidden, unconscious meanings and motifs that are encoded in the dream.

The technique of dream interpretation requires analyzing the manifest content of the dream and deciphering the latent content through various associations and interpretations. This is usually done in a therapeutic setting, where the patient is encouraged to talk freely about their dreams. The therapist helps to examine the patient's own associations and to interpret possible symbols.

One of the cornerstones of this approach is the assumption that dreams often serve as a kind of wish fulfillment. They represent repressed desires and desires that cannot be lived out in the waking state. At the same time, dreams often include mechanisms such as disguise, distortion, and displacement, which serve to make the trauma or unconscious desire more bearable for the conscious mind.

Another important aspect is the role of dream symbols. Freud identified a variety of symbols that can have universally similar meanings, such as phallic symbols or representations of water as metaphors for birth or sexuality. However, he also emphasized the subjective nature of individual symbols, which are strongly dependent on the individual context of the dreamer.

Dream interpretation can also play a role in modern psychotherapeutic approaches beyond classical psychoanalysis, for example in Gestalt therapy, cognitive behavioral therapy or Jungian analysis. Carl Gustav Jung developed his own theories on dream interpretation, in which he placed a stronger focus on archetypal images and the collective unconscious. In Gestalt therapy, on the other hand, dreams can serve as a starting point for creative and experiential processes that encourage the client to playfully explore different aspects of their dreams and integrate them into the waking state.

Duty to provide information

The duty to provide information is a legal and ethical obligation of a psychotherapist to inform patients comprehensively, clearly and comprehensibly about relevant aspects of their treatment. This concept is of outstanding importance in psychotherapy, as it is directly linked to the patient's right to self-determination and autonomy.

The essential information that must be provided as part of the obligation to provide information includes the diagnosis, the proposed therapy methods, possible alternatives, the expected prospects of success and the potential risks and side effects of the treatment. In addition, the therapist must also provide information about the expected costs and duration of the therapy.

The information must be provided in a way that the patient can understand in order to make an informed decision about his treatment. This means that the therapist must refrain from using technical jargon or explain it accordingly and must present complex terms in simple, clear terms.

Another aspect of the duty to provide information is to obtain the patient's consent. Only after the patient has been fully informed can he or she give informed consent to the treatment. This consent can be either verbal or written, depending on the legal requirements of each country or the specific situation.

A special focus is on the principle of "informed consent", also known as informed consent. The patient must not only be informed, but also understand this information and voluntarily agree to it. This includes that the patient can ask questions at any time and have them answered before giving their consent.

In addition, in special cases, such as minors or persons who do not have full legal capacity, there are special regulations and requirements for the culture of education. As a rule, legal guardians or legal representatives must be involved here.

The obligation to provide information does not end with the start of therapy. Rather, it is a continuous process in which the therapist must inform the patient at all times about new findings and changes in the therapy plan. In the event of any significant change in therapy, be it a change in methods or a new diagnosis, the patient must be informed again.

Last but not least, the duty to provide information also serves to build trust between therapist and patient. A well-informed patient feels respected and taken seriously, which strengthens the therapeutic relationship and thus also promotes the success of the therapy.

Dyslalia/articulation disorder

Dyslalia, also known as articulation disorder, refers to a language development disorder in which a person has difficulty forming or articulating sounds correctly. This difficulty often affects preschoolers and can come in various forms. The challenge lies in producing certain speech sounds correctly and thus ensuring the intelligibility of the spoken language.

Articulation disorders can have different causes. They are often due to anatomical deviations, such as cleft palate, misaligned teeth or difficulties in tongue mobility. Neurological disorders or muscular weaknesses in the mouth area that affect motor skills can also play a role. In addition, hearing problems or impairments can also lead to children or adults not perceiving speech sounds sufficiently perceptively, which in turn makes it difficult to form sounds correctly.

In the course of their development, children can have different forms of articulation disorder. The most common types include:

1. **Phonological disorders**: The difficulty here is not so much in the motor execution of the sounds, but in the mental idea of how words should sound. For example, children confuse sounds or omit them.
2. **Articulation disorders in the narrower sense**: This includes the incorrect pronunciation of specific sounds, such as the lisp of 's' and 'z' (sigmatism), or difficulties with sounds such as 'r' (r) or 'k' and 'g' (Kappazism).
3. **Dysglossia**: A rarer form caused by structural or organic abnormalities in the mouth, jaw, or nose.

The treatment of dyslalia is usually carried out as part of speech therapy. Various techniques and exercises are used with the aim of improving motor skills in the mouth area and training correct vocalization. Particularly important here is the recognition and conscious perception of the faulty sounds as well as their gradual correction under the guidance of an experienced therapist.

Depending on the severity and cause of the disorder, a comprehensive diagnostic clarification and an interdisciplinary approach may be necessary. Speech therapists often work closely with dentists, orthodontists, ENT doctors and, if necessary, neurologists to ensure the best possible therapy planning.

Dyssomnias

ABCDEFGHIJKLMNOPQRSTUVWXYZ

Dyssomnias include a group of sleep disorders that are primarily associated with the quantity, quality, or timing of sleep. This category of disorders is particularly relevant in psychotherapy because it interferes deeply with an individual's daily life and well-being, often interacting with other mental and physical health problems.

Insomnia

One of the most common forms of dyssomnia is insomnia, which is characterized by difficulty falling asleep, staying asleep, or waking up early in the morning. Those affected often complain of non-restorative sleep, which leads to impairments in daytime functioning, such as reduced attention, irritability and general fatigue. Both short-term and chronic insomnia can be triggered and maintained by stress, mental disorders such as depression and anxiety, as well as unfavorable sleeping habits and environments.

Hypersomnia

In contrast to insomnia is hypersomnia, which is characterized by excessive sleepiness during the day. People with this disorder do not feel refreshed despite sufficient nighttime sleep and have a strong need to nap during the day. This can significantly affect professional performance and social interactions. Hypersomnia can be primary or secondary to other medical or psychiatric conditions, such as obstructive sleep apnea or major depressive disorder.

Circadian sleep-wake rhythm disorders

These disorders affect the body's internal biological clock, the so-called circadian rhythm. A misalignment of the sleep-wake cycle with the environment, such as shift work or jet lag, leads to sleep discomfort and daytime sleepiness. The most important forms include delayed sleep phase syndrome, in which the individual sleep-wake cycle is shifted backwards, and advanced sleep phase syndrome, in which it is shifted forward. People with circadian sleep-wake rhythm disorders often have difficulty meeting their social and professional obligations, which causes additional emotional stress.

Parasomnias and their distinction

It should be emphasized that dyssomnias must be distinguished from parasomnias. Parasomnias include abnormal events that occur during sleep, such as sleepwalking or nightmares, but these do not primarily affect the quality or quantity of sleep.

Diagnostics and treatment

The diagnosis of dyssomnias is typically made by detailed medical history, sleep diaries and occasionally polysomnographic examinations. Cognitive behavioral therapy, sleep hygiene education and, in some cases, pharmacological interventions play a central role in therapy. The goal is not only to alleviate the symptoms, but also to identify and treat the underlying causes and sustaining factors.

Dysthymia

Dysthymia, also known as persistent depressive disorder, is a chronic form of depression characterized by a long-lasting, depressed mood. This disorder differs from episodic depressive episodes in its persistence and duration. While major depressive disorder often occurs in clearly defined episodes, dysthymia can persist for years, often uninterrupted.

The symptoms of dysthymia are less intense than those of major depressive disorder, but they are also distressing and significantly impair quality of life. Typical features of dysthymia are a depressed mood on most days for at least two years (in adolescents and children over one year), as well as at least two of the following symptoms:

1. **Changes in appetite:** Either decreased or increased appetite.
2. **Sleep disorders:** difficulty falling asleep, difficulty sleeping through the night or excessive need for sleep.

3. **Lack of energy:** Exhaustion and low energy, which makes everyday tasks difficult.
4. **Low self-esteem:** A persistent feeling of worthlessness or inadequate self-judgment.
5. **Difficulty concentrating:** Difficulty concentrating or making decisions.
6. **Feeling of hopelessness:** Pessimism and lack of confidence about the future.

Dysthymia often develops gradually, although those affected and their environment may not recognize it for a long time. Many who suffer from dysthymia become accustomed to the feeling of chronic depression, which makes the disorder part of their "normal state".

The causes of dysthymia are varied and include a mixture of genetic, biological, environmental and psychological factors. A family history of depression can increase the risk, as can chronic stress, traumatic experiences, or ongoing interpersonal problems.

As with other depressive disorders, various therapeutic approaches can be useful for dysthymia. Cognitive behavioral therapy (CBT) is a common treatment method that examines and changes negative thought patterns and behaviors. Other psychotherapeutic approaches, such as interpersonal therapy, which aims to improve interpersonal relationships, can also be helpful. Drug treatments, especially the use of antidepressants, can also be effective in some patients, often in combination with psychotherapy.

The long-term nature of the disorder often requires a persistent and comprehensive treatment strategy that takes into account both the psychological and social aspects of the sufferer's life. It is essential that those affected and their relatives have patience and understanding, as the treatment of dysthymia is a continuous process that requires time and dedication.

Eating disorder

An eating disorder is a complex and often serious mental illness characterized by abnormal eating behaviors and associated thoughts and emotions. These disorders affect diet and eating habits in a negative way and can have significant health consequences, both physical and psychological.

There are several types of eating disorders, including anorexia nervosa, bulimia nervosa, and binge eating disorder, among others.

Anorexia nervosa is characterized by extreme food restriction, an intense fear of weight gain and a distorted body image. Sufferers often have a greatly reduced body weight and tend to meticulously monitor food and calories, often accompanied by excessive exercise.

Bulimia nervosa manifests itself in repeated episodes of overeating (binge eating), followed by compensatory behaviors such as vomiting, excessive use of laxatives, or excessive physical activity. People with bulimia nervosa often experience a sense of loss of control during binge eating and suffer from a strong sense of guilt or shame.

Binge eating disorder is characterized by repeated episodes of overeating, without the subsequent compensatory measures that occur in bulimia nervosa.

Those affected often eat large quantities in the absence of hunger and often experience shame or disgust afterwards.

The treating psychotherapeutic staff takes a multidisciplinary approach to eating disorders, often in close cooperation with doctors and nutritionists. Psychotherapy, especially cognitive behavioral therapy (CBT), has a central position in treatment. The goal is to address the underlying emotional and psychological issues that underlie disordered eating behaviors, while promoting healthy eating habits and a positive body image.

There are many factors that can contribute to the development of eating disorders. Family dynamics, genetic predisposition, socio-cultural pressures, individual psychological aspects such as perfectionism or low self-esteem and stress often play a role. Counselling and education within the family and the wider social environment are also essential components of the therapeutic approach.

Echopraxia

Echopraxia describes the compulsive, involuntary imitation or imitation of other people's movements. This condition often occurs in conjunction with certain neurological or psychiatric disorders, including schizophrenia, Tourette's syndrome, and other conditions that affect the brain's motor control system.

First of all, it is helpful to understand that echopraxia is not simply the conscious decision to imitate another person's movement, as can be the case with social imitation in everyday life. Rather, it is an uncontrolled, often automatic behavior that cannot be voluntarily controlled or suppressed by the affected person.

Echopraxia can occur in a variety of situations, most often when the affected person observes others. For example, someone who suffers from this disorder can automatically imitate the gesture of a counterpart when they brush their hair behind their ear or cross their arms. This can be socially difficult, as the unintentional imitation can be perceived as inappropriate or alienating.

The cause of echopraxia can be traced back to disturbances in the mirror neurons. Mirror neurons are special nerve cells that are activated when someone observes an action and when they themselves perform a similar action. In people with echopraxia, there may be dysregulation in this system, leading to compulsive imitation.

In addition to the neurological component, the psychosocial environment plays a role. Symptoms can be more acute in stressful or socially challenging situations, which can further impair social interaction. Likewise, the intensity and frequency of echopraxia can vary over the course of disorders that are subject to episodic fluctuations, such as schizophrenia.

Treatment for echopraxia focuses primarily on the underlying condition. In cases of schizophrenia, antipsychotic drugs may help, while Tourette's syndrome uses a combination of pharmacological and behavioral therapeutic approaches. It may also be useful to use behavioral therapies to develop alternative, less disruptive ways of responding to triggering situations.

When working with patients, it is important to explain to them that this imitation does not happen consciously and that they have no control over it. This can reduce feelings of guilt and strengthen self-acceptance. Relatives and friends should be informed about echopraxia so that misunderstandings are minimized and a supportive environment is created.

Ego disorder

The term "ego disorder" comes from the field of psychiatry and psychotherapy and describes conditions in which basic functions and boundaries of the ego are impaired or suspended. This includes phenomena in which patients feel that their self, thoughts or physical integrity are disturbed, altered or no longer exist at all. This condition can occur in many ways and depends heavily on the subjective experience of the patient. It is particularly discussed in schizophrenic psychopathology.

The ego disorder encompasses several facets that affect the experience and perception of one's own self:

   1. **Derealization and depersonalization:**

Derealization describes the feeling that the environment seems unreal, alien or artificial. Depersonalization, on the other hand, refers to the experience of feeling oneself alien or detached. Those affected have difficulty perceiving themselves as an independent, consistent person.

   2. **Thought inspiration and thought deprivation:**

Patients experience thoughts that are not recognized as their own, but are perceived as being input or manipulated from the outside. Sometimes they also report that thoughts are withdrawn from them, i.e. that thoughts are suddenly gone or blocked without feeling that they have control over them themselves.

3. Thought propagation:

This is the feeling that one's thoughts are accessible to others or that they can "read" one's thoughts. It is a particularly stressful form of ego disorder, which is often accompanied by a strong paranoia.

4. Ego-boundaries loss:

Here, the boundaries between one's own self and the outside world become blurred. Those affected can no longer clearly assign physical sensations or emotions to their own self or to someone else's.

5. Altered body perception:

A disturbed body perception can lead to body parts being perceived as changed, foreign or absent. This can also occur in the context of depersonalization experiences.

6. Changed sense of time:

The subjective experience of time can also be affected. Patients often report an altered sense of time, in which time either seems to stand still or passes unusually quickly.

The causes of an ego disorder can be manifold. They often occur in the context of schizophrenia, but can also occur in other psychotic disorders, severe depression or as a result of traumatic experiences. The exact mechanisms are not yet fully understood, but a complex interplay of neurobiological, genetic and psychosocial factors is assumed.

In psychotherapy, dealing with ego disorders is particularly challenging. Therapeutic approaches often aim to strengthen the ego and help patients to better integrate their experiences. Various methods such as talk therapy, cognitive behavioral therapy, but also creative therapies are used.

Elective Mutism

Elective mutism, also known as selective or situational mutism, is a complex, psychologically induced communication disorder that usually occurs in early childhood. Children with elective mutism are able to speak and understand normally, but choose not to speak in certain social situations or towards certain people. The phenomenon is not due to a search for attention, but is often an expression of a deep-seated psychological conflict or a significant anxiety disorder.

Children with this disorder, for example, talk to close family members at home, but fall completely silent in school or public contexts. This condition can have a significant impact on social, school and family areas of life, as silence prevents the child from maintaining social relationships, actively participating in lessons or expressing himself in public.

The causes of elective mutism are manifold and not fully understood. However, it is assumed that a mixture of genetic predispositions, temperament traits such as anxiety or shyness, and environmental influences play a role. It often turns out that affected children grow up in families in which high demands are placed on perfection and social competence, or in which a certain overprotection prevails. Traumatic experiences can also be considered triggers.

In the diagnosis, attention is paid to the clinical appearance. Other possible causes of silence, such as developmental disorders, autism or severe speech disorders, must be ruled out. A thorough medical history, supplemented by psychological and medical tests if necessary, is crucial here.

Psychotherapeutic treatment of elective mutism usually requires a multimodal approach. Behavioral therapy methods have proven to be particularly effective in helping the child overcome the fear of speaking in certain situations. This is often done in small, controlled steps (graduated exposure). Systemic approaches that involve family and school can also be helpful. In some cases, drug treatments are also considered, especially in the case of severe generalized anxiety.

A central component of therapy is the establishment of a trusting relationship between the therapist and the child. Through positive reinforcement and targeted exercises, communicative competence and self-confidence are to be gradually increased. The involvement of parents and teachers in the therapeutic process is also of great importance in order to ensure constant support of the child in various areas of life.

EMDR (Eye Movement Desensitization and Reprocessing)

EMDR (Eye Movement Desensitization and Reprocessing) is a psychotherapeutic method that has been specially developed for the treatment of post-traumatic stress disorders. Originally conceived by the American psychologist Francine Shapiro in the late 1980s, this form of therapy has since experienced extensive validation and acceptance in both theoretical and practical terms.

The core idea of EMDR is based on the assumption that stressful experiences and traumas are blocked in neuronal processing and cannot be correctly integrated into long-term memory. These unprocessed memories can later serve as a source of mental disorders such as post-traumatic stress disorder (PTSD), anxiety disorders or depression.

In the EMDR therapy process, clients are guided to focus on traumatic memories while also following horizontal eye movements initiated and controlled by the therapist. Alternatively, other bilateral stimuli, such as tactile stimulation (e.g. alternating tapping on the hands) or auditory stimuli, can also be used. This dual attention approach is intended to help process the blocked memories and lead to adaptive resolution.

EMDR therapy follows a structured approach divided into eight phases:

1. **Anamnesis and treatment planning:** In this phase, the relevant life history events and traumatic experiences of the client are recorded. The therapist identifies specific memories and current triggers that are relevant to EMDR processing.

2. **Client preparation:** In this phase, the client is informed about the EMDR process, and coping strategies are taught to help deal with potentially emerging stressful memories.
3. **Assessment:** The therapist helps the client select specific memories and identify the different components of these memories, such as images, negative cognitions, emotions, and physical sensations.
4. **Desensitization:** The client focuses on the traumatic memory and performs the eye movements at the same time. Bilateral stimulation is continued until the strain decreases significantly or disappears completely.
5. **Installation:** In this phase, positive cognition is linked to the original traumatic memory to promote integration into adaptive understanding.
6. **Body test:** This checks whether there are still physical tensions or sensations associated with the traumatic memory. These will then be further processed.
7. **Conclusion:** The therapist ensures that the client is emotionally stable and teaches coping strategies for everyday life.
8. **Re-evaluation:** In this phase, the client's progress is reviewed and it is determined if further sessions are needed or new traumatic memories need to be worked on.

EMDR is a dynamic and intensive process that can achieve significant improvements in trauma patients both in the short term and in the long term. The method has proven its effectiveness in many clinical studies and is recognized by numerous professional associations, such as the American Psychological Association (APA), as an empirically based form of therapy.

Emotional Intelligence

Emotional intelligence refers to a person's ability to recognize, understand, discern and use their own emotions as well as the emotions of other people. This competence affects both intrapersonal and interpersonal skills and plays a crucial role in the way individuals respond to their environment and interact with others.

Emotional intelligence includes various aspects such as self-confidence, self-regulation, motivation, empathy and social skills. Self-awareness involves understanding one's emotions and how those feelings influence thoughts and actions. People with high self-awareness recognize their emotional states, are aware of their strengths and weaknesses, and can precisely evaluate how their emotions affect those around them.

Self-regulation describes the ability to control impulsive reactions and to control stressful emotions in a targeted manner. This makes it possible to remain calm and balanced in stressful situations. Self-regulation strategies include techniques such as breathing exercises, meditation, and cognitive restructuring that help individuals mitigate negative emotional effects.

Motivation in the context of emotional intelligence refers to how intrinsic and extrinsic factors can be used to promote goal-directed behavior. People with high emotional intelligence are often able to maintain their passion for long-term goals and use their emotions to continuously motivate themselves, even when they encounter obstacles.

Empathy is the ability to recognize and empathize with other people's emotions. This makes it possible to cultivate interpersonal relationships, understand conflicts and offer support. An empathic individual perceives nonverbal cues and can integrate them into interactions with others, allowing for deeper and more meaningful connections.

Finally, social skills encompass the wide range of competencies necessary for effective interactions and collaboration with others. This includes communication skills, conflict resolution, influence, and leadership skills. People who are socially competent can easily build and maintain networks and act appropriately and effectively regardless of the social or professional environment.

Emotional intelligence is not static, but can be further developed through targeted practice and reflection. Many therapeutic approaches, such as cognitive behavioral therapy or mindfulness-based interventions, aim to strengthen emotional intelligence by helping individuals develop a deeper understanding of themselves and others. This can improve well-being, strengthen resilience and make interpersonal communication more effective.

Empathy

Empathy is the ability and willingness to empathize with and understand the feelings, thoughts and perspectives of another person. In psychotherapy, empathy is one of the basic competencies that enables the therapist to build a trusting and supportive relationship with his clients.

Empathy differs from mere pity or compassion in that it encompasses not only the perception and recognition of emotions, but also empathy and the active effort to explore and comprehend the inner world of the other. It is crucial that the therapist gives space to the client's feelings and accepts them in a non-judgmental and respectful manner.

There are different dimensions of empathy: Cognitive empathy refers to the ability to understand another person's thoughts and intentions and take their perspective. Emotional empathy, on the other hand, involves the actual empathy and empathy of the other's emotions. These two aspects are interconnected and reinforce each other to allow for a deeper connection and better understanding.

A high level of empathy on the part of the therapist significantly promotes the therapeutic process. It allows the client to feel safe and understood, which in turn increases the willingness to open up and show emotional vulnerability. This is especially important because many clients are confronted with deep-rooted fears, traumas, or emotional blockages in therapy that require a certain amount of openness and trust.

Empathy in therapeutic practice requires a high degree of mindfulness and presence. The therapist must listen actively, attentively observing non-verbal signals such as body language and facial expressions of his client and being able to react to subtle emotional nuances. The therapist must also be able to assess and dose one's own emotional resonance in order to maintain professional distance and at the same time remain authentic and compassionate.

In addition, empathy plays a central role in modulating interventions and therapeutic techniques. An empathic therapist is better able to recognize when it is appropriate to ask a certain question, use a technique, or intervene in a certain way. This increases the effectiveness of the therapy and supports the client in gaining insights and experiencing positive change.

Endocrinology

Endocrinology is a medical specialty that deals with the endocrine glands and their hormone production, as well as the hormonal regulatory mechanisms of the body. Endocrine glands, such as the thyroid gland, adrenal glands, pancreas, pituitary gland, and gonads (ovaries and testicles), release hormones directly into the blood. These hormones serve as messenger substances that control and regulate various bodily functions.

Hormones play an essential role in regulating metabolic processes, growth and development, water and electrolyte balance, reproduction, and response to stress. A disturbance in the endocrine system can therefore have far-reaching effects on the entire organism and lead to a wide variety of clinical pictures. Such disorders can affect both an overproduction (hyperfunction) and an underproduction (hypofunction) of hormones.

Diagnostics in endocrinology usually include blood and urine tests to determine hormone levels, imaging techniques such as ultrasound or MRI to visualize the glands, and functional tests that check the response of the glands to certain stimuli. The common clinical pictures that are examined and treated in endocrinology include diabetes mellitus, thyroid diseases (such as hyperthyroidism or hypothyroidism), Addison's disease, Cushing's disease, polycystic ovary syndrome (PCOS) and hormonal growth disorders.

In psychotherapeutic practice, endocrinology can offer important interfaces, as hormonal imbalances are often accompanied by psychological symptoms. For example, thyroid diseases can trigger depressive moods or anxiety. Chronic stress can lead to dysregulation of the hypothalamic-pituitary-adrenal (HPA) axis, which in turn can cause psychological and physical symptoms. Therefore, a sound understanding of the endocrinological basis is important for psychotherapists in order to provide holistic care to patients and to develop interdisciplinary approaches to treatment.

Enkopresis

Encopresis, also known as defecation, is a disorder characterized by repeated voluntary or involuntary excretion of stool in places not intended for it, such as clothing or floors. This behavior occurs in a child who has already reached the age at which bowel control is normally developed, usually from the age of four. The diagnosis of encopresis requires that the disorder occurs at least once a month over a period of at least three months.

There are two main forms of encopresis: primary encopresis, in which the child has never achieved complete bowel control, and secondary encopresis, in which the child begins to defecate again after a period of clean bowel control.

Encopresis can have both organic and psychological causes. Organic causes include chronic constipation followed by faecal incontinence, in which hardened stool remains in the intestine and more liquid stool comes out around it. From a psychological point of view, various factors can contribute to encopresis. Emotional stress, family conflicts, traumatic experiences or other mental disorders such as anxiety and depression can play a significant role. In addition, a disturbed toilet education or a negative experience regarding going to the toilet can further exacerbate the problem.

Treatment options for encopresis include a combination of medical and psychological interventions. Medically, laxatives or stool softeners can be administered to alleviate constipation and promote normal bowel behavior. An important aspect of treatment is also the establishment of regular toilet times and a positive reinforcement of correct toilet behavior.

Depending on the underlying causes, behavioral therapy approaches, family therapy or depth psychology-oriented therapies can be used psychotherapeutically. The aim is to strengthen the child's self-esteem, reduce fears and clarify any family conflicts. Parents and caregivers play a central role in the treatment process and are usually actively involved in therapy to learn supportive measures and create a conducive environment for the child.

Enuresis

Enuresis is a urological and often psychological disorder characterized by involuntary urination during the day and/or night. This disorder occurs mainly in children, but can also persist in adolescence and adulthood. It is divided into two main types: primary enuresis and secondary enuresis.

Primary enuresis

This type occurs when a child from the age of five has never achieved bladder control for an extended period of time. The cause of this is often a maturation delay of the central nervous system, which means that the child is unable to effectively perceive and respond to the signals of a full bladder. Genetic factors also play an important role, as enuresis often runs in families.

Secondary enuresis

This form of enuresis occurs when a child has been dry for at least six months and then suddenly starts wetting again. Secondary enuresis can be triggered by various stressors, such as family conflicts, separation or loss, as well as special medical conditions such as urinary tract infections or diabetes mellitus. Psychological factors, including emotional distress and mental health issues, also often contribute to its development.

Diagnosis

The diagnostic clarification is carried out by means of a comprehensive anamnesis and physical examination. Parents and caregivers are asked in detail about the frequency and timing of wetting. In addition, urine samples and ultrasound examinations may be necessary to rule out organic causes. Psychological assessments can be helpful in identifying possible emotional and psychological triggers.

Therapy

The treatment of enuresis is multimodal and based on the individual needs of the affected child. Therapeutic approaches include:

- **Behavioral therapies**: Techniques such as bell machine training, in which the child is woken up by an alarm as soon as he starts wetting, can be very effective.
- **Drug therapy**: In certain cases, desmopressin-containing medication may be prescribed to reduce nocturnal urine production.
- **Psychotherapy**: If psychological factors play a role, individual or family therapies can be helpful. Here, the emotional stability of the child and family dynamics are worked on.
- **Bladder training**: Techniques to strengthen bladder control through targeted exercises and behavior-based methods can improve urination behavior.
-

Prognosis

Most children grow out of enuresis without long-term problems, especially if proper therapy is initiated. Continued support and patience from parents and carers are crucial to promote the child's self-esteem and well-being during treatment. In the long term, very few children develop persistent problems if they are treated in a timely and adequate manner.

Epigenetics

Epigenetics refers to the scientific study of the mechanisms by which environmental factors and life events influence gene activity without causing changes in the DNA sequence itself. In psychotherapy, knowledge of epigenetic processes is of great importance because it provides a deeper understanding of how experiences and environmental conditions can influence a person's mental health and behavior, even across generations.

Epigenetic changes occur mainly through chemical modifications of the DNA or histone proteins around which the DNA wraps. Two of the most important epigenetic mechanisms are DNA methylation and histone modification. DNA methylation involves binding a methyl group (CH_3) to DNA, which often leads to the silencing of genes. Histone modifications involve chemical changes to the histone proteins that modify the structure of chromatin, thereby facilitating or complicating access to certain genes.

In psychotherapy, it is central to understand that epigenetic markers can be influenced by a variety of factors, including traumatic experiences, chronic stress, diets, environmental toxins, and social support systems. Such influences can not only change individual gene expression, but can also be inherited. For example, studies have shown that traumatic experiences can cause epigenetic changes in parents that are passed on to their offspring, indicating a kind of "memory" of environmental conditions in the genetic material.

This has far-reaching implications for the understanding of mental disorders and their treatment. Therapeutic interventions can be specifically aimed at altering the conditions that promote negative epigenetic patterns. Stress management programs, therapeutic recreation of safe and supportive environments, and targeted nutrition and lifestyle interventions can help promote adaptive epigenetic changes and support long-term mental health changes.

The finding that epigenetic mechanisms play an important role in gene expression regulation opens up new perspectives on the plasticity of the human genome in response to psychological interventions. This poses a challenge for therapists, who must consider these complex mechanisms in their understanding and practice in order to provide comprehensive support to patients. Knowledge of epigenetics can help the therapist create more personalized and potentially effective treatment plans that not only target the symptoms, but also address deeper, causative factors.

Erickson, Milton

Milton H. Erickson (1901-1980) was an American psychiatrist and psychotherapist who is considered one of the most influential figures in modern hypnotherapy. His work and methods have had a profound impact on the understanding and application of hypnosis and psychotherapy.

Erickson's approach is based on the belief that the unconscious is a positive and creative force that can be used to heal and well-being an individual. He was known for his non-directive and patient-centered techniques and emphasized the importance of personalized therapies tailored to the client's unique needs and resources.

One of his outstanding methods was utilisation, in which he took up spontaneous behaviours, comments or symbols of the client and constructively integrated them into the therapeutic process. This technique illustrates his flexible and creative approach to hypnotherapy, where he often used everyday situations or seemingly irrelevant details to bring about therapeutic change.

Erickson's work was informed by a number of principles, including the idea that every person is capable of finding their own solutions to their problems. He often used indirect suggestions and stories, so-called metaphors or analogies, to awaken and promote the resilience and creative potential of his clients.

His hypnosis techniques have often been described as non-traditional, as they deviated from the formal, directive methods of his time. Erickson was sometimes able to put his clients in trans-like states by giving them simple but individually tailored suggestions. This was often referred to as "gentle hypnosis", and it made it possible to use the natural processes of thinking and experiencing to bring about changes in behaviour and perception.

Another notable feature of his approach was his ability to use mimesis – observing and mirroring his client's behavior to build a therapeutic alliance. This technique helped to build trust and collaboration, which facilitated the therapeutic process.

Erickson's influence extends far beyond hypnotherapy and has influenced many psychotherapeutic schools and techniques, including neurolinguistic programming (NLP) and short-term therapy. His writings and case studies are still valuable to scholars and practitioners today, as they offer a wealth of insights and techniques that continue to inspire new generations of therapists.

He presented a variety of concepts and inspiring ideas that have had a lasting impact on the psychotherapeutic landscape. In doing so, he expanded the understanding of the healing power of the unconscious and showed how creative and flexible approaches in therapy can bring about profound changes.

Existential therapy

Existential therapy is an approach within psychotherapy that focuses on the fundamental questions and challenges of the human condition. This form of therapy emerged from existential philosophy, especially from the works of thinkers such as Søren Kierkegaard, Friedrich Nietzsche, Jean-Paul Sartre and Viktor Frankl. Its central concern is to accompany and support people in their existential questions and needs.

Existential therapy explores the elementary aspects of human life, such as freedom, responsibility, isolation, meaning and finiteness. Instead of focusing primarily on symptom relief, she strives for a deeper examination of her clients' existential concerns. The focus is on the question of the meaning of life and the authentic shaping of one's own existence.

For therapeutic practice, this means an encounter at eye level, in which the therapist does not appear as an expert, but as an equal companion on the way to greater self-understanding and individual fulfillment. The client is encouraged to explore themselves and their values, to acknowledge their own responsibility and to make personal decisions in a self-determined way.

An essential aspect of existential therapy is the encounter with one's own mortality. By viewing death as an inevitable part of life, therapy allows clients to develop a deeper appreciation of the present moment and the time they have left. This confrontation can help to reduce fears and support a more authentic lifestyle.

In the therapeutic relationship, great importance is attached to authenticity and presence. The therapist does not offer ready-made solutions, but supports the client in finding his own answers. Various methods are used to promote self-reflection and awareness of one's own existence. This includes conversations, creative forms of expression and other interventional techniques that are tailored to the client's individual situation.

The goal of existential therapy is not only to improve the quality of life, but also to lead a deeper, self-determined lifestyle based on authentic values and convictions. It helps clients understand the nature of their existential worries and create a more fulfilling and meaningful life in the face of these worries.

Expansion of consciousness

Expansion of consciousness is a multidimensional concept in psychotherapy that involves the expansion of an individual's perception and thought processes. The aim is to enlarge the spectrum of subjective experience and to make deeper layers of consciousness accessible. This often includes increased mindfulness and an intensified experience of one's own inner and outer world.

In a therapeutic context, expansion of consciousness can be achieved through various methods and techniques. These include meditative procedures, breathing exercises, hypnosis, psychedelic therapy and other forms of self-awareness. These methods aim to bring the client into contact with previously unconscious aspects of their being, which often allow for deep insights and transformative experiences.

Meditative methods such as mindfulness meditation promote the expansion of consciousness by systematically directing attention to the present moment. This helps to break through automated patterns of thought and behavior and opens up new perspectives and deeper self-reflection. Breathing exercises and body-centered methods can also facilitate access to expanded states of consciousness by intensifying the connection between body and mind.

Hypnosis uses trance states to expand the client's consciousness. In these trance states, access to unconscious thoughts, emotions and memories is easier to access. This allows problematic patterns to be identified and worked on that are difficult to access in the normal state of consciousness.

Of particular note are psychedelic therapies, which allow clients to experience profound changes in their perception and emotional state through the controlled use of mind-altering substances such as psilocybin, MDMA, or LSD. These substances can bring issues deeply rooted in the unconscious to the surface and enable intensive psychotherapeutic work that holds the potential for significant therapeutic breakthroughs.

The effects of the expansion of consciousness are manifold. They can include an increased understanding of one's own life situation, deeper emotional integration, an improved sense of self-efficacy and an overall improved quality of life. However, these processes often require careful therapeutic support in order to responsibly navigate possible challenges and risks.

In psychotherapy, the expansion of consciousness is considered a powerful tool that can be tailored to individual needs and therapeutic goals. It supports transformation and enables clients to develop a more comprehensive understanding of themselves and their environment.

Exposure method

The exposure method is a central method in behavioral therapy, which was specially developed to help patients overcome their anxiety and avoidance behaviors. The core of the exposure procedure is to confront the patient in a targeted and repeated manner with the situations, objects or thoughts they fear, without any actual dangers or negative consequences. This takes place in a controlled and therapeutically supported environment.

When the exposure procedure is carried out, a hierarchy of anxiety-inducing stimuli is often created. This hierarchy helps to make the confrontation gradual and systematic, starting with mild anxiety triggers and ending with highly stressful ones. The patient is thus gradually introduced to the anxiety-triggering situation and learns that the feared consequences either do not occur at all or are less serious than originally assumed.

There are different forms of exposure: in vivo exposure, which takes place directly in the real environment, and in sensu exposure, in which the patient merely imagines the anxiety-provoking situations. Both methods have proven to be effective, although the choice of method depends on the individual needs and specific problems of the patient.

Another important element of the exposure procedure is the duration of the confrontation. The exposure should last long enough for the patient to have the opportunity to experience habituation, i.e. a decrease in the fear reaction. Through repeated and prolonged exposure, the patient becomes increasingly desensitized to the object of fear or the situation.

A commonly used model for exposure is systematic desensitization, which also involves a gradual, gradual approach to the dreaded stimuli, often accompanied by relaxation techniques to reduce physiological arousal. Another model is the flooding technique, in which the patient is directly and intensively confronted with the strongest fear stimulus in order to abruptly reduce the fear response.

The goal of exposure therapy is to enable the patient to have new learning experiences and thus transform the cognitive and emotional aspects of anxiety. The patient learns that his fear is exaggerated or unfounded and that avoidance behavior is rather counterproductive in the long run. By reducing anxiety and avoidance, an increase in quality of life and an improvement in functioning in everyday life can be achieved.

In the therapeutic process, the accompaniment and support of the patient is of great importance. The therapist not only provides guidance and structure, but also emotional support and encouragement. Cognitive behavioral therapy techniques are also often incorporated to identify and modify dysfunctional thought patterns that contribute to the maintenance of anxiety.

The exposure method is particularly effective in the treatment of anxiety disorders such as phobias, panic disorders and post-traumatic stress disorder, but is also successfully used for obsessive-compulsive disorder and other mental illnesses.

Expressive speech disorder

An expressive language disorder, also known as expressive language development disorder, is a communicative disorder that specifically refers to a person's ability to produce language and express verbal messages effectively. This disorder affects both oral and written language and can occur in different contexts and ages, with a particularly common diagnosis in children.

People with an expressive language disorder have difficulty formulating their thoughts, ideas, feelings and needs in a clear and understandable way. They may have limited vocabulary and often find it difficult to find words or form sentences that conform to grammatical rules. This applies to language production as well as linguistic syntax and sentence structure.

Symptoms of this disorder vary greatly and can take on mild to severe manifestations. Children may have difficulty constructing complete sentences or tell stories that are disjointed or difficult to understand. You could also make simple grammatical mistakes, such as omitting important words or using incorrect verb forms.

The causes of expressive language disorder are diverse and can include both genetic and environmental factors. Possible genetic influences can include familial predispositions to language and communication disorders. Environmental factors could include insufficient language stimulation in early childhood or other developmental conditions.

This disorder is usually diagnosed through a comprehensive linguistic and psychological evaluation, which includes both standardized tests and observations. The aim of this evaluation is to identify the specific language deficits and to distinguish them from other potential disorders such as receptive language disorders or general developmental delays.

The treatment of an expressive speech disorder usually requires targeted speech therapy, which is carried out by a speech therapist. Therapeutic approaches can be individualized and include techniques to expand vocabulary, consolidate grammatical structures and improve narrative skills. Close collaboration with parents and teachers is often necessary to support the child's progress in more natural communication environments and to maximise the applicability of the skills learned.

Long-term prognosis for individuals with an expressive language disorder may vary depending on the severity and timing of the start of the intervention. Early and continuous speech therapy can significantly help improve communication skills and thus also increase the chances of academic and social success.

Family constellation

Family constellation, also known as systemic constellation, is a psychotherapeutic method that is used to explore and solve emotional and psychological problems. It was developed by Bert Hellinger and is based on the principle that individuals often adopt unconscious patterns and dynamics within their family that influence their current life circumstances and relationships.

The process of family constellations usually begins in a group setting, but individual constellations are also possible. The client, who is referred to as a "constellation leader", selects representatives from the group to represent members of his family or essential aspects of his problem. These representatives are then intuitively positioned in the room so that they reflect the relationships and interactions within the family system.

The representatives often report physical sensations, emotions or movement impulses that they perceive in the assigned places. These phenomena are referred to as the "knowing field" or "morphogenetic field" and provide insights into hidden or unresolved conflicts in the family. The therapist who leads the constellation supports this process with targeted questions and observations, which reveal hidden dynamics and relationships.

A central element of the family constellation is the illustration of systemic entanglements, such as unconscious loyalties, feelings of guilt and shame or the adoption of other people's fates. By making these entanglements visible, the client can develop new perspectives and gain understanding for deep-rooted patterns.

The therapist guides participants to interventions, often involving symbolic actions or phrases, to initiate new orders and healing movements in the system. These changes often lead to a positive change in the client's perception and relationship patterns.

Finally, the constellation is reflected on and the client is given the opportunity to integrate the experienced insights into his everyday life. Family constellations can trigger profound emotional processes, which is why it is important that they are carried out by experienced and trained therapists.

The method is not only used in psychotherapy, but is also used in other areas such as coaching, supervision and counselling to shed light on systemic relationships in organisations or teams. Nevertheless, the primary goal of the family constellation remains the clarification and healing of individual and family systems through the recognition and release of unconscious dynamics and entanglements.

Family history

The family history is an indispensable part of the diagnostic phase in psychotherapy and describes the systematic collection and analysis of the medical, psychological, social and cultural history of a family. It serves to gain a comprehensive understanding of the family influences and dynamics that may contribute to the development and maintenance of mental disorders.

The collection of the family history is carried out through a structured conversation in which the psychotherapist asks specific questions in order to gather information about past and present health and illness conditions of the family members. Particular attention is paid to mental illnesses, such as depression, anxiety disorders, addiction problems or schizophrenia. Physical diseases that could have a genetic component, such as diabetes, cardiovascular disease or cancer, are also of interest.

In addition, the family history also considers psychosocial and cultural factors. These can be family role models, communication patterns, coping mechanisms as well as traumatic events such as divorces, deaths, violence and abuse. The influence of cultural norms and values, as well as migration-related experiences, is also captured, as these can have a significant impact on mental health.

Another central element of family history is genogram creation, a visual representation of the family structure over several generations. A genogram helps to better identify and understand relationships and patterns, such as recurring conflicts or transferences. Conclusions can also be drawn about transgenerational trauma, i.e. inherited traumatic experiences.

The quality of the family history depends crucially on the accuracy and openness of the data collected as well as the therapist's ability to create a trusting atmosphere of conversation. It requires a sensitive and respectful approach to be able to talk about stressful and intimate topics. It is important to identify and appreciate not only the pathological aspects, but also the resources and strengths of the family.

The information obtained from the family history is incorporated into the diagnostic assessment and therapy planning. They help to individualize the therapeutic approach and develop targeted interventions. For example, systemic approaches such as family therapy may be appropriate if it turns out that family interactions contribute significantly to the problem.

Family Therapy

Family therapy is a form of psychotherapy that aims to improve interactions and relationships within a family system. It is based on the belief that problems and behaviors of individuals must be considered and understood in the context of their family relationships. Instead of focusing only on the individual, family therapy involves all relevant members of the family unit in the therapy process.

A central assumption of this form of therapy is that the family is an interdependent system. This means that changes in one part of that system, such as one individual, inevitably have an impact on the other parts of the system. Therefore, it makes sense to involve all members in the therapeutic process in order to achieve sustainable change.

The sessions can take place with the whole family as well as in smaller subgroups. The most common goals include improving communication with each other, resolving existing conflicts and strengthening understanding for each other. Various therapeutic techniques and methods are used. For example, role plays, structured exercises or systemic constellations can be used to make the dynamics in the family system visible and changeable.

In family therapy, the therapist plays a facilitator role, asking questions and sharing observations to guide family members to a better understanding of their interactions. The therapist helps the family identify patterns and dynamics that may be contributing to problems. Through these insights, the family can develop strategies to improve their relationships.

Typical problems treated in family therapy include relationship problems between parents and children, marital problems, communication difficulties, behavioral problems in children and adolescents, addiction problems, as well as dealing with grief and loss.

Another important concept of family therapy is the Multigenerational Model, which was developed by Murray Bowen. It looks at family problems in the context of family history over several generations. It analyzes how recurring behavioral patterns and emotional reactions are passed on, and how they affect the current problems of the family.

Solving family problems and promoting positive change can greatly improve the quality of life for all family members and build supportive, loving relationships. Family therapy can help create lasting change by providing a deep and comprehensive understanding of family relationships.

Fight-or-flight

The term "fight-or-flight" refers to the physiological reaction of the body to situations perceived as threatening. This response, also known as the "fight-or-flight response," is triggered by the autonomic nervous system, specifically by activating the sympathetic nervous system. This leads to the release of stress hormones such as adrenaline and norepinephrine.

When a person perceives danger, the body either prepares to fight the threat or flee from it. This is an evolutionarily developed survival mechanism that has played a crucial role in human history by enabling rapid responses to imminent dangers.

The physical changes initiated by the fight-or-flight response are many and include:

Increasing heart rate to pump more blood to muscles

Dilation of the bronchi to improve oxygen uptake

Releasing glucose from energy reserves to provide energy quickly

Slowing down of non-critical bodily functions such as digestion and peristaltic movements of the intestine

Increase in blood clotting to minimize blood loss in the event of injury

Psychologically, the state of peak arousal prepares the mind to make quick and potentially life-saving decisions. Attention is strongly focused on the threat, while the perception of the environment is narrowed.

In modern society, the fight-or-flight response also takes place in stressful situations that are not life-threatening, such as professional pressure or interpersonal conflicts. This can lead to chronic stress, which can cause various health problems, including heart disease, mental disorders such as anxiety and depression, and sleep disorders.

In therapeutic sessions, we often dedicate ourselves to the task of identifying the triggers of the fight-or-flight response and developing methods to manage these responses in a meaningful way. Cognitive behavioral therapy (CBT) techniques, mindfulness training, and relaxation techniques are effective interventions to help patients better control physiological and psychological responses to stress.

Since the fight-or-flight response is deeply rooted in our biology, understanding and working with this mechanism in a targeted manner is an essential tool in psychotherapy.

Flow

The term "flow" refers to a special mental state that is described as an optimal state of experience. This state is often reached when a person is fully immersed in an activity that they find intrinsically motivating and challenging at the same time. The Hungarian-American psychologist Mihály Csíkszentmihályi coined the term and researched its characteristics and prerequisites.

An essential characteristic of the flow state is the complete absorption in the current activity, with the awareness of time, fatigue and even basic needs such as hunger and thirst receding into the background. People who are in the flow often report a strong sense of control over their actions and decisions, as well as a deep satisfaction and joy while performing the activity.

The conditions for experiencing flow include several central aspects: First, the activity should have a clear goal so that the person knows exactly what is expected of them. Second, immediate feedback is important so that the person can continuously adapt and improve their actions. Thirdly, the task in question must have a balance between one's own abilities and the difficulty of the task – too little challenge leads to boredom, too much challenge leads to frustration.

Flow can be experienced in a variety of contexts, whether it's sports, making music, writing, or even doing a job. This state not only promotes individual well-being, but also personal development and performance. In therapeutic practice, the experience of flow can be specifically promoted in order to give clients access to positive experiences and self-efficacy experiences.

The concept of flow is not only important in the field of self-help and personal development, but is also used in positive psychology and organizational psychology. In therapy, it can be used to help clients identify activities that have the potential to induce flow experiences, thus helping to improve quality of life and overall well-being.

In summary, flow is a state characterized by intense and pleasurable engagement in an activity and promoted by specific conditions. This condition has far-reaching positive effects on individual experience and behavior and is therefore a valuable concept in the context of psychotherapy.

Framing

In psychotherapy, framing refers to the way in which information, events or experiences are presented and structured in order to promote certain meanings, interpretations or emotional reactions in clients. This concept originated in communication and social psychology, but is often used in therapeutic practice to influence or change a client's perception and behavior.

A significant aspect of framing is that people construct their reality based on the interpretation and context of the information. These constructions are not neutral, but are shaped by linguistic and contextual frames (frames). For example, the same state of affairs can be perceived differently depending on whether it is seen as an "opportunity" or a "problem".

In therapeutic practice, framing can be used to change entrenched thought patterns and their emotional reactions. For example, a therapist might reframe a client's tendency to see failures as completely negative events by presenting them as valuable learning experiences. This can help the client develop a more flexible and positive outlook and improve their coping strategies.

Another value of framing in therapy is to shift the client's focus from negative to positive aspects of a situation. Suppose a client has difficulties in interpersonal relationships and tends to focus on the negative interactions. The therapist could reframe these situations by making the client aware of the successful interactions and the possibilities for improving relationships. This can boost self-esteem and create hope.

Framing also plays a crucial role in changing beliefs and behavioral patterns. A well-known example is cognitive behavioral therapy (CBT), where framing or reframing dysfunctional thoughts leads to a change in negative emotions and behaviors. A therapist might help a client who believes they are always clumsy in social situations by looking for examples where the client has successfully mastered social interactions and offering them as a new framework.

During the framing process, language is of central importance. The choice of words, the emphasis on certain aspects of a statement, and the context in which information is presented can greatly influence interpretation and emotional resonance. Many therapeutic schools, such as narrative therapy, use targeted linguistic framing to transform the client's individual story and self-perception.

Freud, Sigmund

Sigmund Freud was an Austrian neurologist and the founder of psychoanalysis, an influential method for researching and treating mental disorders. Born in 1856 in the Austro-Hungarian city of Freiberg, Freud initially devoted himself to neurology, but then developed a deep interest in psychopathology through his work with mentally ill patients. His theories and techniques revolutionized the understanding of the human mind and continue to shape psychotherapy today.

Freud's work focused on the concept of the unconscious, which he considered to be a central site of our psychic lives. He postulated that many of our thoughts, feelings and memories are hidden in the unconscious and influence through various mechanisms – such as repression or sublimation – affecting our behavior and mental health.

A core part of his theory was the tripartite division of the human psyche into the id, ego and superego. The id stands for the unconscious drives and desires that are shaped by primitive and hedonistic impulses. The ego represents the conscious mind that tries to mediate between the impulsive demands of the id and the moral and social norms of the superego. The superego, in turn, embodies the moral conscience and values formed by upbringing and social influences.

Another crucial theory of Freud was his concept of psychosexual development, according to which the human personality is formed through several stages of development: oral, anal, phallic, latent and genital phases. For Freud, each phase was linked to specific conflicts that, if not successfully resolved, can lead to later psychological problems. This assumption led to the idea that many neurotic symptoms can be traced back to early childhood experiences and unresolved conflicts.

In practice, Freud developed the technique of free association, in which patients are encouraged to speak freely about their thoughts and feelings in order to uncover hidden conflicts and repressed memories. Dream interpretation also played a central role in Freud's therapeutic approach; he considered dreams to be the "royal road to the unconscious" and believed that they offered essential insights into a person's unconscious desires and conflicts.

Freud's influence on psychotherapy and culture as a whole can hardly be overestimated. Although his theories and methods have often been criticized and further developed, they continue to form the basis for many modern psychotherapeutic approaches and have inspired new fields of research such as depth psychology and psychodynamics.

Although some of his ideas are considered outdated today, Freud's contribution to psychology remains essential for understanding complex psychological processes and developing treatments that provide deeper insights into human consciousness. In this respect, Freud is a key figure in the history of psychotherapy and a central personality for anyone who wants to deal with the inner mechanisms of the human mind.

Further education

In psychotherapy, the term "continuing education" refers to the ongoing process in which already trained and licensed psychotherapists continuously expand, deepen and update their professional skills, knowledge and competencies. This process is essential to meet the high standards of professional practice, to integrate new findings and methods of psychotherapy research, and to meet the ever-changing needs and developments in the field of mental health.

A continuing education measure can take various forms, including seminars, workshops, professional conferences, supervisions, case studies and specialised courses. These events are often organized and carried out by renowned professionals, institutes or professional associations. They provide a platform to present and discuss innovative approaches and therapeutic techniques, thus promoting the exchange of knowledge and practical experience.

Continuing education includes not only learning new therapeutic approaches and techniques, but also reflecting on one's own therapeutic practice and modifying existing methods. It contributes to the personal and professional development of the therapist and supports him in critically questioning and improving his own strengths and weaknesses. Topics such as ethics, intercultural competence and working with special target groups can also be part of the training, as they make an important contribution to the quality of therapeutic work.

In addition, continuous training is a prerequisite for quality assurance in psychotherapy. Many professional associations and legal regulations prescribe a minimum amount of annual training in order to maintain the license as a psychotherapist. This guarantees that therapists always stay up to date with the latest science and practice and can offer their clients the best possible support.

The specific content and scope of the training can vary depending on the subject area, individually set priorities and professional goals. Some therapists specialize in certain forms of therapy such as behavioral therapy, depth psychology, systemic therapy or other methods as part of their further training. Others expand their skills with regard to certain disorders or patient groups, such as trauma, eating disorders or children and adolescents.

Generalized anxiety disorder

Generalized anxiety disorder (GAD) is a widespread mental condition characterized by persistent and excessive anxiety that extends to a wide variety of areas of life. Those affected experience an almost constant worry, which is often perceived as uncontrollable and occurs more often than it is justified by concretely threatening situations. This form of anxiety differs from normal everyday fears in terms of its duration and intensity.

Symptoms of generalized anxiety disorder include a variety of both cognitive and physical ailments. On a cognitive level, there is constant worry, nervousness, difficulty concentrating, and a feeling of being overwhelmed. Physical symptoms can manifest themselves in muscle tension, trembling, sweating, palpitations, gastrointestinal problems and sleep disorders.

The diagnosis of this disorder follows the criteria of the Diagnostic and Statistical Manual of Mental Disorders (DSM-5) or the International Classification of Diseases (ICD-10). The disorder must persist for a period of at least six months and significantly interfere with daily activities. In addition to the diagnostic criteria, a thorough differential diagnosis is also required to rule out other mental or physical conditions that could cause similar symptoms.

The causes of GAD are diverse and can include genetic, biological, and psychosocial factors. A family history, neurobiological mechanisms and personal life events such as chronic stress or traumatic experiences potentially contribute to the development of the disorder. People with a certain neurotic temperament or those who have difficulty tolerating insecurities seem to be particularly vulnerable.

There are a number of effective approaches to treating generalized anxiety disorder. Cognitive behavioral therapy (CBT) is considered an extremely effective method. It aims to identify and change dysfunctional thought patterns and behaviors. This is done through techniques such as cognitive restructuring and exposure to fearful situations. Relaxation techniques and mindfulness training are often used as supplementary measures.

Drug treatment options include selective serotonin reuptake inhibitors (SSRIs) and serotonin-norepinephrine reuptake inhibitors (SNRIs), which are often considered the first choice in pharmacotherapy. In some cases, benzodiazepines or other anti-anxiety drugs may also be used for a short time, but caution should be exercised because of the risk of developing dependence.

A multidisciplinary therapeutic approach that combines psychotherapy, drug treatment and psychosocial support has proven to be particularly successful. In addition to individual therapy, group therapy can also be helpful in finding social support and reducing isolation through exchange with other sufferers.

In the long-term perspective, treatment aims to reduce symptomatic distress, strengthen coping skills, and improve quality of life. Through comprehensive and individualized therapy, many sufferers can learn to deal with their fear and lead a fulfilled life.

Geriatric Psychotherapy

Geriatric psychotherapy is a specialized area of psychotherapy that deals with the mental health of older people. It takes into account the specific challenges and life circumstances associated with aging. This includes both physical and psychological changes that often occur at this stage of life.

A central aspect of geriatric psychotherapy is coping with losses. Many older people are confronted with the loss of life partners, friends and family members. These losses can cause deep grief and loneliness. In addition, the decline in physical abilities, such as mobility and sensory functions, often requires adaptation to new life circumstances and can affect self-esteem.

Cognitive changes are another important topic of geriatric psychotherapy. Age-related cognitive impairment can range from mild memory loss to severe dementia. Therapy may include techniques aimed at maintaining cognitive performance and provides support in adapting to these new challenges.

In addition, the treatment of chronic pain plays an important role. Pain management and coping with physical discomfort that often comes with age are essential components of therapy. In this context, close cooperation with medical professionals is often sought in order to ensure holistic care.

Social isolation and loneliness are also central issues addressed in geriatric psychotherapy. Older people are more likely to experience social isolation, which can significantly affect their mental health. Therapeutic interventions can aim to strengthen social networks and promote opportunities for participation in social life.

An important part of geriatric psychotherapy is also the recording and processing of life reviews. Reflecting on one's own life, dealing with past experiences and integrating these experiences into one's present self-image can pave the way to a feeling of meaning and contentment in life.

Therapeutic methods in geriatric psychotherapy range from cognitive behavioral therapies to talk therapies to creative-therapeutic approaches such as art or music therapy. Each method is tailored to the individual needs and circumstances of the patient.

In addition, it is essential to emphasize interdisciplinary work. Geriatric psychotherapy often works closely with other disciplines, including gerontology, medicine, nursing, and social work, to ensure comprehensive care.

Finally, the training and support of relatives plays a decisive role. Relatives and caregivers are involved in the therapeutic process to inform and support them about the challenges and needs of the elderly.

Gestalt therapy

Gestalt therapy is a holistic approach within psychotherapy that was developed in the 1940s and 1950s by Fritz Perls, Laura Perls and Paul Goodman. It is based on humanistic psychology and places special emphasis on the here and now, personal responsibility and becoming aware of feelings, thoughts and behavioural patterns.

A central aspect of Gestalt therapy is the emphasis on the present and immediate experience. Instead of delving deep into the patient's past, therapy focuses on what is happening in the moment. The aim is to help patients become aware of and fully accept their current experiences in order to enable change and growth. The exploration and awareness of one's own emotions and thoughts is in the foreground in order to recognize entrenched patterns and blockages.

Another important principle of Gestalt therapy is the idea of a self-regulating wholeness. Therapy sees individuals as complex systems that are in constant interaction with their environment. This interplay is described as a figurative process in which individual aspects or "figures" (thoughts, feelings, memories) emerge from the overall picture or "background" of the experience and disappear again. A person's ability to consciously and authentically experience and influence this process is considered an integral part of their mental health.

Gestalt therapy often works with special techniques and exercises to support the therapeutic process. A well-known method is the "empty chair" or "chair dialogue", in which the patient imagines that a certain person or aspect of themselves is sitting on an empty chair in front of them and has a dialogue. This technique aims to gain access to unprocessed feelings and thoughts and enables direct confrontation with them.

An essential element of Gestalt therapy is also the emphasis on mindfulness and awareness. Patients are encouraged to closely observe and describe their sensory perceptions, emotions, and physical sensations without judging or analyzing. Through this increased mindfulness, unconscious processes can be brought into consciousness and better understood.

The goal of Gestalt therapy is not only to alleviate symptoms, but also to enable the patient to lead an authentic and self-determined lifestyle. By promoting self-awareness and inclusive thinking, patients are to be empowered to identify and pursue their own needs and desires. This provides the possibility of a more fulfilling, creative and healthy life.

Group therapy

Group therapy is a therapeutic method in which a small group of people work together on their psychological, emotional or social problems, under the guidance of one or more trained therapists. This form of therapy offers participants the opportunity to address interpersonal problems and learn from each other in a protected and supportive environment.

The composition of the group can be based on various criteria, for example according to specific diagnoses such as depression, anxiety disorders, addiction problems or post-traumatic stress disorder. There are also groups that cater to specific age groups or life situations, such as young adults, the elderly, or people in separation and divorce situations. A typical group size is between 6 and 12 people, which creates a sufficiently intimate atmosphere, but at the same time offers enough variety of perspectives and experiences.

A central element of group therapy is the exchange between the group members. By sharing their own experiences and listening to the experiences of others, participants develop a better understanding of their own problems and often find that they are not alone in their concerns. These interactions can help strengthen social skills and learn new, healthier behaviors. The mechanisms of group dynamics, such as the emergence of trust and solidarity, also play a major role in the therapeutic process.

The therapist acts as a moderator and supports the group by promoting communication processes, providing assistance with reflection and, if necessary, initiating therapeutic interventions. The aim is to steer the exchange constructively and, if necessary, to use therapeutic techniques. The therapist also makes sure that each participant has enough space to express his or her concerns and that conflicts that arise in the group are dealt with productively.

Another important point of group therapy is the so-called group-specific process, in which a certain dynamic and a common path develop in the course of the sessions. This gives participants the opportunity to try out behaviors directly and receive feedback from the other group participants. In this way, they can gain new insights and recognize and change existing patterns.

The duration of group therapy can vary and ranges from a few weeks to several years. The sessions usually take place weekly and last about 90 minutes. The long-term success of group therapy depends largely on the regularity and consistency of participation as well as on the openness and willingness of each individual to self-reflection and change.

Habituation

Habituation is a fundamental psychological and neurobiological phenomenon that can be observed in both humans and animals. It describes the gradual reduction of the willingness to react to a repeatedly presented stimulus. This process occurs when an organism reacts progressively less to a stimulus that has been recognized as safe and non-threatening.

In the context of psychotherapy, habituation plays an essential role, especially in the treatment of anxiety disorders and phobias. Here, the client is repeatedly confronted with the anxiety-inducing stimulus in a systematic and controlled manner, in a procedure known as exposure therapy. Through this controlled and step-by-step approach, the client can learn that the anxiety-inducing stimulus is not actually as dangerous as it was originally assumed. Over time, the fear response is reduced, and the client can develop a neutral or even positive attitude towards the stimulus.

At the neurobiological level, habituation is explained by repeated activation of neuronal circuits in the brain. With each repetition of the stimulus, synaptic connections seem to react less strongly because the stimulus is recognized as less significant. This saves the brain energy and resources by minimizing unnecessary reactions to non-threatening stimuli.

In addition to anxiety therapy, habituation is also used in other therapeutic contexts. In pain therapy, for example, repeated exposure to a non-harmful pain stimulus can cause the patient to react less intensely to it.

Another area where habituation is relevant is how to deal with sensory overload in neurodivergent individuals, such as people with autism spectrum disorders. Here, tolerance can be built up through repeated and controlled exposure to certain stimuli, which helps those affected to better cope with everyday sensory overload.

In behavioral medicine, habituation is used to reduce maladaptive behavior patterns. A smoker who gradually gets used to the stimulus of cravings can learn that the craving for a cigarette decreases after some time if he does not give in to this craving immediately.

Hallucinations

Hallucinations are perceptual-like experiences that occur without an external stimulus and are perceived by those affected as real sensory events. Hallucinations play a central role in psychotherapy, especially in the diagnosis and therapy of psychotic disorders, as they often occur in connection with mental illnesses such as schizophrenia, bipolar disorder and severe depression.

There are different types of hallucinations that differ in sensory modalities. These are:

Auditory hallucinations: The affected person hears voices or sounds that are not present. They often report voices that make comments, insult them or give orders. Auditory hallucinations are the most common form and are particularly common in schizophrenia.

Visual hallucinations: Here, people see things that don't exist, such as people, animals, or flashes of light. This type of hallucination is common in neurodegenerative diseases such as dementia, but also in intoxication.

Olfactory and gustatory hallucinations: These affect the sense of smell and taste. Those affected perceive strange or unpleasant smells and tastes that are not present. This form occurs less frequently, but can be an indication of neurological disorders.

Tactile hallucinations: In this case, people experience touch, tingling or movement on or under the skin without any physical stimulus. This type of hallucination can occur in the context of substance abuse, especially cocaine or alcohol.

Hallucinations can occur episodic or persistent and vary greatly in intensity and frequency. Hallucinations are often extremely stressful for those affected and can lead to considerable suffering. They have a significant impact on the social, professional and private lives of those affected.

Treatment of hallucinations is usually multimodal. Psychopharmacological approaches, especially the use of antipsychotics, are in the foreground to reduce the intensity and frequency of hallucinations. In addition, psychotherapeutic methods are used, such as cognitive behavioral therapy, which can help those affected to learn how to deal with hallucinations and better cope with their symptoms.

An understanding of the individual triggers and the significance of the hallucinations in the patient's life is often helpful. Therapeutic interventions may also include psychoeducational approaches to raise awareness of the condition and develop strategies for dealing with stress and negative emotions that can potentially increase hallucinations.

Heller's dementia

Heller's dementia, also known as childhood disintegrative disorder or Heller's syndrome, is a rare neuropsychiatric disorder that usually occurs in children aged 3 to 4 years who have previously shown normal development. It was first described at the beginning of the 20th century by the Austrian pediatrician Theodor Heller.

This disorder is characterized by a dramatic and seemingly sudden loss of previously acquired abilities. This loss affects several areas of child development, including language, social skills, play, motor skills, and self-help skills.

In detail, Heller's dementia manifests itself in a regressive course that can last for about 6 to 12 months. Changes that have begun can manifest themselves in a decline in the ability to interact socially. Children lose their learned ability to communicate appropriately with their environment and relatives. Linguistically, there can be a huge decline, up to a complete loss of language skills after they have already been developed.

In addition to linguistic and social regression, interest in playful and imaginative activities is often reduced. Another characteristic feature is the decline in the child's independent abilities. Previously acquired motor skills and self-care skills, such as dressing and eating independently, can also be significantly impaired.

Diagnostically, it is crucial to differentiate Heller's dementia from other neuropsychiatric disorders such as autism spectrum disorders. The striking difference lies in the previous normal development and the sudden loss of abilities, which is not observed in most autistic children.

The causes of this disorder are not yet fully understood, but it is believed that genetic, neurological, and environmental factors may play a role. When looking at the neurological and biological components, some studies show evidence of structural and functional abnormalities in the brains of affected children.

The treatment of Heller's dementia requires a multidisciplinary approach, which usually includes a combination of speech therapy, occupational therapy, behavioral therapy and, if necessary, drug therapy. The goal of therapy is to restore lost abilities as much as possible and to develop new coping strategies to improve the quality of life of the affected children and their families.

Histrionic personality disorder

Histrionic personality disorder (HPS) is a mental disorder characterized by a deep-rooted pattern of emotionally exaggerated and attention-seeking behaviors. People with HPS strive to be the center of attention and often exhibit dramatic, theatrical behavior to achieve this goal. This can be done through flashy clothing, lively gesticulation, excessive emotional reactions, and the constant search for recognition and validation.

A central feature of histrionic personality disorder is the need for constant validation and admiration. Sufferers tend to perceive relationships as closer or more intimate than they actually are, and often engage in inappropriately seductive or provocative behavior to get the attention of others. Their emotional expressions are often superficial and changeable, which can lead to their relationships remaining superficial and lacking depth.

Another characteristic of HPS is the excessive preoccupation with external appearances and the desire to attract attention through appearance and behavior. These individuals are welcome to take on the role of the victim or portray themselves as a dramatic hero to gain sympathy and support. Their emotional behavior, including expressions of sadness or joy, can seem overly dramatic and inappropriately intense.

In social situations and relationships, people with HPS often seek praise, recognition, and affection and are sensitive to criticism or rejection. This tendency can cause them to struggle to maintain long-term and stable relationships. Their desire to be the center of attention can sometimes make other people feel overwhelming or manipulative.

Although the exact causes of histrionic personality disorder are not fully understood, it is believed that a combination of genetic, biological, and environmental factors play a role. Some studies suggest that early experiences, such as inconsistent parenting or excessive attention and pampering, could contribute to the development of this disorder.

The treatment of histrionic personality disorder is usually done through psychotherapy, with the aim of strengthening self-esteem and improving the way people deal with feelings. Therapeutic approaches, such as cognitive behavioral therapy (CBT), can help identify and change dysfunctional thoughts and behavioral patterns. A trusting therapeutic relationship is crucial to allow patients to experience real emotional intimacy and improve their interpersonal skills.

The prognosis for people with HPS varies, depending on the severity of the disorder and commitment to therapy. With the right support and therapeutic intervention, sufferers can learn to reduce their attention-seeking behaviors and have healthier, more stable relationships.

Holy Seven (after Alexanders)

The "Holy Seven" according to Franz Alexander are seven emotional conflicts that have been identified as potential roots of psychosomatic illnesses. The term "Holy Seven" alludes to the apparent sacredness and immutability of these conflicts, as Alexander formulated them in his theory of psychosomatic medicine.

At the heart of the theory is the assumption that certain psychosocial stressors and emotional conflicts can cause specific organic diseases. Alexander, an important representative of psychosomatics and psychoanalysis, developed this list as a kind of catalogue of mental stress that can lead to physical symptoms and illnesses.

The seven conflicts are:

1. **Anxiety:** The threat of external or internal sources of danger can lead to chronic stress and thus to physiological changes. Fear, as a recurring aspect of life, has the ability to put the entire organism in a state of alert.
2. **Frustration:** Ongoing frustration due to unmet needs or blocked goal achievement can create emotional and physical tension, which can manifest itself in various physical ailments.
3. **Aggression:** Suppressed or misdirected aggression can express itself on a physical level, especially if there is no adequate outlet for these emotions. The body may react with symptoms ranging from muscle tension to stomach ulcers.
4. **Guilt:** Feelings of guilt and shame can be deep-seated emotional conflicts that lead to constant inner

stress and subsequently to various psycho-physiological disorders.
5. **Loneliness:** Social isolation and feelings of loneliness have far-reaching consequences for physical and mental health. The lack of social interactions can contribute to both depression and physical ailments.
6. **Separation:** Experiences of loss through death, divorce or other forms of separation from significant people have the potential to leave behind psychological trauma that can be reflected physically.
7. **Sexual conflicts:** Unfulfilled sexual desire, feelings of guilt about one's own sexuality or problems in sexual relationships are profound emotional conflicts that often manifest themselves psychosomatically.

The conceptual framework of the "Holy Seven" forms a bridge between mental and physical health. The hypothesis is that each of these types of conflict causes specific biological reactions in the body that can lead to manifest diseases over time. Franz Alexander emphasized the need to address these deep-seated emotional causes in psychotherapy in order to promote long-term healing and holistic well-being.

His work has laid the foundation for modern psychosomatic approaches and raised awareness of the fact that behind many physical ailments there are often unresolved emotional conflicts. The holistic view of body and soul, as expressed in Alexander's theory of the "Holy Seven", remains an integral part of psychotherapeutic practice and psychosomatic medicine.

Humanistic Therapy

Humanistic therapy represents an important branch within the psychotherapeutic landscape and is deeply rooted in the philosophical concepts of the humanist movement. It emerged in the 1950s and 1960s as a reaction to the then dominant theories of behaviorism and psychoanalysis, which were perceived as too deterministic and reductionist.

The core of this therapeutic direction is the image of the human being, which considers the human being to be fundamentally good and with a natural urge for self-realization and autonomy. It emphasizes that each person is a unique individual and has the potential to live a full and meaningful life. The basic assumption is that mental health problems result when this potential is inhibited by unfavorable environmental conditions or negative life experiences.

A central concept of Humanistic Therapy is the self-actualization tendency, a term that was significantly coined by Carl Rogers. This tendency describes the inherent drive of every human being to develop, grow and fully exploit their potential. Another important concept is that of "congruence," which describes the state in which a person's self-image coincides with their actual experiences.

The role of the therapist in Humanistic Therapy is to create a supportive, non-directive environment that enables the client to independently reach insights and find solutions. The therapist is seen more as a companion and less as an advisor. The focus is on the present and the future rather than the past, unless this is considered necessary to understand current problems.

A key feature of this form of therapy is the emphasis on the therapeutic relationship, which is often considered the heart of the healing process. The relationship is characterized by three main components:

1. **Empathy:** The empathy of the therapist who tries to see the world through the eyes of the client.
2. **Unconditional positive appreciation:** The acceptance and appreciation of the client without judgment.
3. **Authenticity:** Authenticity and transparency of the therapist.

Well-known humanistic approaches and methods are client-centered conversational psychotherapy according to Carl Rogers, Gestalt therapy according to Fritz Perls and existential therapy according to Rollo May and Viktor Frankl. Client-centered conversational psychotherapy focuses on creating a climate in which the client feels safe enough to talk openly about his or her thoughts and feelings. Gestalt therapy focuses on the here and now and the client's awareness of his or her current thoughts, feelings and actions. Existential therapy examines deeper questions of human existence such as freedom, responsibility and finding meaning.

Humanistic therapy also emphasizes creative forms of expression and body-oriented approaches. Techniques such as role-playing, creative expressions such as painting or writing, and body-oriented procedures provide clients with ways to externalize and better understand internal processes.

The effectiveness of Humanistic Therapy is particularly evident in the treatment of disorders associated with low self-esteem, interpersonal problems and existential crises. By fostering self-acceptance, personal responsibility, and authenticity, clients can often experience significant change in their lives.

By prioritizing human potential and the need for self-actualization, Humanistic Therapy offers a profound and respectful way to promote mental health and support individual change.

Hyperkinesia

In psychotherapy and medicine, hyperkinesis refers to an abnormality that is characterized by excessive and uncontrollable movements. The term is made up of the Greek words "hyper" (over) and "kinesis" (movement). This motor disorder can occur in different forms and have a wide variety of causes.

In many cases, hyperkinesis is manifested by excessive motor activity, which can manifest as constant movement, fidgeting, rocking, or involuntary muscle twitching. The movements are often not targeted and can occur both at rest and during targeted activities. Affected individuals have difficulty controlling their body movements, which can lead to restrictions in everyday activities.

Hyperkinesis can occur as a symptom of various neurological or mental illnesses. One of the most well-known forms of hyperkinesis is hyperactivity, which is often observed in connection with attention deficit hyperactivity disorder (ADHD). In ADHD, affected children or adults are not only hyperactive, but also show other symptoms such as inattention and impulsivity.

Diseases such as Tourette's syndrome or Huntington's disease can also cause hyperkinesis. In Tourette's syndrome, hyperkinesis manifests itself in the form of tics, which are manifested by rapid, repetitive and involuntary movements or vocalizations. Huntington's disease is a neurodegenerative disease in which people experience uncontrollable, dancing movements.

The diagnosis of hyperkinesis requires a thorough medical history and careful examination by specialists or therapists. In addition to physical examinations, neuropsychological tests and imaging techniques are often used to identify possible underlying causes.

Treatment depends on the cause of hyperkinesis. In cases of ADHD, therapeutic measures such as behavioral therapy, psychoeducation and drug treatment can be used. In neurological diseases such as Tourette's syndrome or Huntington's disease, the focus is often on drugs that aim to reduce involuntary movements. Occupational therapy and physiotherapy can have a supportive effect by teaching people techniques to better control their movements.

Hypersomnia

Hypersomnia, also known as excessive daytime sleepiness, refers to a condition in which a person feels an unusually strong need for sleep during the day. This excessive sleepiness can occur despite sufficient night's sleep and often leads to those affected unintentionally falling asleep in inappropriate or inappropriate situations. Hypersomnia can significantly affect daily life and is often associated with reduced performance and quality of life.

The symptoms of hypersomnia can be diverse. Those affected often report a constant feeling of fatigue, which persists even after sleeping for a long time. This persistent fatigue can lead to difficulty concentrating, memory problems, and a general slowdown in cognitive processes. In addition, the social and professional life of those affected can be significantly affected, as the constant need for sleep leads to problems in the performance of everyday tasks.

In the field of diagnostics, hypersomnia is first evaluated clinically through a detailed anamnesis interview, in which sleep habits, sleep quality and possible accompanying symptoms are asked. Often, objective sleep studies, such as polysomnographic measurements or the Multiple Sleep Latency Test (MSLT), are also carried out to accurately record sleep architecture and sleepiness. Particular care is taken to rule out other sleep disorders, such as sleep apnea or periodic movement disorders.

The causes of hypersomnia are diverse and can be both organic and psychological. Organic causes include neurological disorders such as narcolepsy, certain hypothalamic pathologies or sleep apnea. Psychological causes can include severe depressive episodes, anxiety disorders or chronic stress. Drug side effects or the abuse of drugs and alcohol are also suspected of causing hypersomnia.

The treatment of hypersomnia depends on its cause. In the case of primary hypersomnia, which has no specific underlying disease, drug treatment approaches are usually in the foreground. Stimulants such as modafinil or methylphenidate can help increase wakefulness and reduce daytime sleepiness. In the case of secondary hypersomnia that occurs in the context of another underlying disease, treatment focuses on the underlying cause. Psychotherapeutic interventions, especially behavioral therapy, can have a supportive effect and help those affected to develop better sleep hygiene and learn stress-reducing techniques.

Hypnotherapy

Hypnotherapy is a therapeutic technique that uses hypnosis to treat mental and physical problems. In this method, the patient is put into a trance-like state in which the subconscious mind is particularly receptive to suggestions. Hypnosis in itself is a natural state of altered attention or consciousness in which focus is intensified and peripheral perception is reduced.

In a therapeutic context, hypnosis serves as a tool to promote healing processes and to support behavior change. The hypnotherapist first gently introduces the patient to hypnosis by guiding him or her into a deep but awake state through relaxation techniques or monotonous stimuli. In this state, also known as a hypnotic trance, the patient is often deeply relaxed, but at the same time highly concentrated.

Within this trance, various therapeutic techniques can be used to address specific problems. This includes the use of suggestions, visualizations, and metaphors to influence the patient's subconscious mind and promote positive changes in thoughts, feelings, and behavioral patterns. For example, a patient suffering from anxiety can learn to reevaluate and control their fear responses through guided visualizations and positive suggestions.

Hypnotherapy is often used as part of a broader therapeutic program and can be used in combination with other psychotherapeutic approaches, such as cognitive behavioral therapy or psychodynamic therapy. This integration allows for an individually adapted treatment that takes into account both the conscious and the unconscious aspects of the psychological problem.

A central concept of hypnotherapy is ideomotor activity, in which thoughts and suggestions evoke involuntary physical reactions. For example, the suggestion that an arm becomes light and floats up while the patient is deeply relaxed can actually cause the arm to move. Such reactions are used to deepen and strengthen the therapeutic process.

Over the past few decades, research has proven the effectiveness of hypnotherapy for a wide range of disorders. These include anxiety disorders, depression, pain management, post-traumatic stress disorder (PTSD), somatic complaints and addiction disorders. The possibilities of application are wide-ranging, and hypnotherapy is carried out in individual, group and even online settings.

Fundamental to the success of hypnotherapy is the therapeutic relationship between therapist and patient. Trust and open communication are crucial for the patient to get involved in the hypnosis sessions and allow inner changes. Qualified hypnotherapists provide a safe environment in which patients can explore their deepest fears, worries, and desires.

Hypochondriacal disorder

Hypochondriac disorder, often referred to as hypochondria, is a mental illness in which sufferers are strongly convinced that they are seriously ill despite the lack of medical evidence of an actual physical illness. This belief is often accompanied by intense anxiety and constant worries about one's own health.

People with hypochondriac disorder mistakenly interpret normal physical sensations or minor symptoms as signs of serious illness. For example, a simple headache could be interpreted as a symptom of a brain tumor. This misinterpretation often leads to disproportionate anxiety and can cause significant stress and worry.

A central feature of hypochondriacal disorder is the constant need for medical confirmation and the frequent change of treating physicians. Those affected repeatedly seek medical advice and diagnostic tests, although previous examinations and medical insurance companies have not been able to prove a serious illness. These visits usually offer only short-term reassurance before fears flare up again.

In many cases, patients suffer from great suffering. This can lead to various psychosocial impairments, for example in the ability to work or in social relationships. The focus on the supposed health problems takes up so much space that other areas of life are neglected.

The exact cause of hypochondriac disorder is not fully understood, but it is believed that a combination of genetic, biological, psychological, and environmental factors play a role. Certain personality traits, such as a tendency to be anxious and increased sensitivity to physical sensations, can increase the risk.

In the therapy of this disorder, psychotherapists often use cognitive behavioral therapy (CBT). This form of therapy aims to change the dysfunctional thought patterns and behaviors of patients. Patients learn to question their hypochondriacal fears and to assess their physical sensations more realistically. For some patients, drug treatment, for example with antidepressants, can also be helpful, especially if there are also depressive symptoms or other anxiety disorders.

A successful therapeutic approach requires not only the treatment of acute symptoms, but also preventive measures to prevent relapses. It is important that those affected learn to develop stress management strategies and to find a healthy balance between self-care and a realistic assessment of their health. In many cases, it also makes sense to involve close caregivers in order to create a supportive social environment.

I/Superego

The ego and the superego are two central concepts in classical psychoanalysis, developed by Sigmund Freud. They are integral to understanding the human psyche and its dynamics.

The self

The ego (also referred to as the ego) acts as an intermediary between the external world, the id and the superego. It is able to make rational decisions and supports the individual in adapting to reality. The ego operates primarily on the basis of the reality principle, which states that actions and impulses must be carried out taking into account the environment and its conditions.

The ego is responsible for executive control over thoughts, actions, and emotions. It assesses risks and opportunities, plans actions and sets priorities. Another important function of the ego is the use of defense mechanisms. These psychological strategies serve to cope with fears and inner conflicts by repressing, distorting or transforming unpleasant thoughts and feelings into the unconscious.

The ego develops in early childhood and matures through social interactions, upbringing, and experiences. It tries to find a balance between the often contradictory demands of id, superego and the real world.

The superego

The superego (or superego) represents the moral authority of the personality. It arises from the internalization of parental and societal norms and values. The superego consists of two components: the ego ideal and the conscience.

The ego ideal includes all moral and idealistic aspirations that the individual strives for. It represents the self-image that a person aspires to, including consummate ethical and moral standards. Conscience, on the other hand, is the part of the superego that is responsible for punishing the ego when it violates these internalized standards. It manifests itself in feelings of guilt, shame and inferiority.

The superego aims to monitor and direct the behavior of the individual in order to keep it in accordance with internalized moral and social norms. This can lead to inner conflicts, especially if the id has strong urges and desires that the superego sees as unacceptable.

Interaction between ego and superego

The relationship between the ego and the superego is often characterized by tension. While the ego tries to find realistic and practical solutions, the superego makes moral demands and idealistic demands. This discrepancy can lead to inner conflicts, which the ego tries to cope with through various defense mechanisms.

A well-developed and strong ego is central to mental health, as it has the ability to effectively integrate and manage the various demands of id, superego, and reality. Solutions and compromises that the self finds must be both feasible and morally justifiable, which is often a complex and challenging process.

Through therapy, the understanding and strength of the ego can be promoted, which helps the patient to find a better way of dealing with inner conflicts and external challenges.

ICD-10

The ICD-10, or "International Statistical Classification of Diseases and Related Health Problems, 10th Revision", is a globally recognized classification of medical diagnoses published by the World Health Organization (WHO). This classification serves as a universal diagnostic tool that allows healthcare providers to identify and code diseases, disorders, and health conditions in a standardized way. ICD-10 plays a central role in psychotherapy and psychiatry, as it contains detailed categories for mental disorders and behavioral problems.

This classification is divided into 21 chapters, each covering specific groups of diseases and conditions. Chapter F is particularly relevant for mental and behavioral disorders. It includes categories such as mood disorders (for example, depression and bipolar disorder), anxiety disorders, personality disorders and many other mental disorders. Each of these categories is further divided into more specific diagnoses, allowing for precise and consistent diagnostics.

The structure of the ICD-10 codes consists of an alphanumeric system. A code begins with a letter, followed by two digits and optionally further subcategories separated by periods. For example, major depressive disorder is described by the code F32.x, where "x" stands for specific degrees of severity or manifestations.

For psychotherapists, the ICD-10 is not only an instrument for diagnosis, but also for documentation and communication with other professionals and institutions. By using the ICD-10 codes, they can share their observations and treatment plans in a standardized language that is understood worldwide. This is particularly relevant for research purposes, insurance issues and the development of evidence-based treatment guidelines.

Another important aspect of ICD-10 is that it is regularly updated to reflect new scientific findings and clinical experience. The current version, the ICD-10, has undergone several minor adjustments since its introduction to improve its accuracy and usefulness.

The ICD-10 also has a social and ethical dimension, as it helps to reduce the stigma of people with mental disorders. By providing a comprehensive and differentiated classification, it helps to promote understanding and acceptance of mental illnesses and to provide appropriate support to those affected.

Illusory misjudgement

Illusionary misunderstanding is a psychological phenomenon in which a person's perception differs from reality, often due to unconscious desires, fears, or conflicts. In psychotherapy, this phenomenon is often understood as a form of defense mechanism in which a person perceives reality in a different or distorted way in order to protect themselves against painful or unpleasant feelings.

A classic example of illusory misunderstanding is when an individual interprets a hostile gesture or statement as friendly because he or she cannot bear the reality of the aggression. This misperception of reality can be applied to external objects as well as to interpersonal interactions.

Illusionary misrecognition differs from other forms of perceptual distortion, such as hallucinations or delusions, in that it is not completely detached from reality. Instead, an actual object or event is misinterpreted or seen in a different light. For example, a person who suffers from illusory misrecognition might hear something significant or threatening in a sound that is just a random background noise.

This phenomenon can be studied on several levels of the psychic apparatus. On the conscious level, illusory misunderstanding can lead to misunderstandings and communication problems. However, on a deeper, unconscious level, it can serve as a defense system that helps the individual deal with internal conflicts and unresolved emotional issues. Illusionary misrecognition can thus be uncovered and analyzed in a psychotherapeutic session in order to understand and resolve the psychological processes behind it.

The therapeutic intervention for illusory misjudgement aims to identify the distortions of perception and to work on the underlying fears and conflicts. This is done through exploratory conversations in which the therapist helps the patient gradually grasp and accept reality. This allows adaptive mechanisms to be activated that allow the patient to deal with his environment in a more realistic and constructive way.

Imagination

Imagination is a central term in psychotherapy and refers to the ability of the human mind to create inner images, scenes, experiences and feelings that are not directly stimulated by the present external reality. This skill is an essential tool for many therapeutic approaches that aim to understand and transform inner processes, emotional states, and personal experiences.

In therapeutic practice, imagination is often used in techniques such as the guided imagination journey, visualization, and working with metaphor-rich scenarios. Through targeted exercises and instructions, clients can evoke inner images that symbolically represent their inner conflicts, fears, desires and needs.

An example of the use of imagination in therapy is the method of the "empty chair technique". This technique is often used as part of Gestalt therapy. Clients imagine that a certain person or an aspect of themselves is sitting on an empty chair opposite them. They then enter into an imaginary dialogue with this "counterpart" in order to work through unresolved conflicts, express emotions and gain new insights.

Imagination can also have a significant effect in the field of trauma therapy. Specific procedures such as the "safe place" technique allow traumatized clients to create a safe and calming place in their minds to which they can mentally retreat when they feel overwhelmed or under stress. This technique helps to improve their emotional regulation and restore a sense of security and control.

The neurobiological basis of imagination shows that similar brain areas are activated as in real perceptions. This illustrates the potentially powerful effect of imaginative techniques, as the brain often perceives imagined experiences as real as they actually experienced. This makes it possible to bring about changes in perception and emotional experience that take place beyond purely rational cognition.

Imagination also plays an important role in art therapy practice. Here, creative-creative imagination is used to make inner processes and conflicts visible and to process them through artistic forms of expression. Clients can create symbolic representations of their inner world through painting, drawing or other creative activities, which can then be interpreted and discussed therapeutically.

Immune system and psyche

The interaction between the immune system and the psyche is a multifaceted and complex topic that deals with the mutual influence of these two systems. This interaction forms the basis of an interdisciplinary field of research called psychoneuroimmunology (PNI). This discipline investigates how emotional and genetic factors, as well as environmental conditions and lifestyle choices, influence the immune system and thus overall health.

The immune system serves as the body's protective mechanism against pathogenic microorganisms such as bacteria, viruses and fungi. It is made up of a variety of cell types and molecules that work together to fight off infection and repair damaged tissue. The most important components of the immune system include white blood cells (leukocytes), antibodies and various cytokines that act as signaling substances between cells.

The psyche encompasses the totality of all conscious and unconscious mental processes. These include emotions, thoughts, beliefs, and attitudes that shape an individual's experience and behavior. Psychological conditions such as stress, anxiety or depression have been shown to have an impact on the immune system. Prolonged stress, for example, can increase the production of stress hormones such as cortisol, which can impair the function of immune cells and increase susceptibility to infections, among other things.

Communication between the psyche and the immune system takes place via various biochemical and neural pathways. Stress hormones such as cortisol and adrenaline, which are released via the hypothalamic-pituitary-adrenocortical axis (HPA axis), play an important role in this. These hormones can modulate the activity of immune cells and affect the balance between the body's pro-inflammatory and anti-inflammatory responses.

The nervous system is also involved in this interaction. Special nerve cells in different parts of the brain, such as the limbic system and the hypothalamus, are able to coordinate immune responses. Neuropeptides and neurotransmitters such as serotonin and dopamine also play a role in bidirectional communication between the brain and the immune system.

Negative emotions and psychological stress can affect the vitality of the immune system, while positive emotional states such as joy and contentment can have a beneficial effect on immune function. Studies have shown that people with strong social ties and a positive emotional background have a better immune response and a lower susceptibility to infections.

Furthermore, psychotherapeutic interventions such as cognitive behavioral therapy (CBT), mindfulness-based stress reduction (MBSR) and other forms of emotional support can help stabilize mental health and thus indirectly strengthen the immune system. By regulating stress and promoting positive coping strategies, such interventions can improve immune function and thus overall health.

Impulse control disorders

Impulse control disorders are characterized by the inability or significant difficulty to resist impulses or urges that may be harmful to the affected person or others. These disorders manifest themselves in different, often specific, behavioral patterns that are different from short-term outbreaks caused by stress and often recur.

One of the most well-known impulse control disorders is intermittent explosive disorder (IED). Individuals with IED exhibit recurrent, disproportionate outbursts of anger or aggressive behavior that is not justified by the situation. These outbursts can involve physical violence or destructive behavior and often occur suddenly without a clearly identifiable trigger.

Another form is kleptomania, in which there are recurrent, uncontrollable urges to steal items that are not done out of financial or personal necessity. Those affected experience a significant increase in tension before the theft and a feeling of relief or satisfaction immediately afterwards.

Pyromania is also one of the disorders of impulse control. In this case, those affected feel the urge to start a fire and feel a strong excitement or euphoria during the act. The act of setting fire does not take place in the context of revenge, financial motives or political convictions, but is experienced as an inner need.

Trichotillomania, or compulsive hair pulling, is another disorder in which sufferers feel an irresistible need to pull out their hair, resulting in visible hair loss. This act is often used as a stress or anxiety management mechanism, although it only brings short-term relief and can lead to shame and social isolation in the long term.

Pathological gambling is likewise an impulse control disorder and is characterized by repeated episodes of problematic gambling that interferes with the sufferer's life in significant areas such as personal health, relationships, and professional performance. Those affected feel a strong inclination to bet or take risks, often accompanied by irrational beliefs about having to win.

Therapeutic approaches for impulse control disorders can include cognitive behavioral therapy (CBT), dialectical behavioral therapy (DBT), or pharmacological interventions. The therapeutic process often focuses on recognizing and understanding the underlying triggers, as well as developing impulse control strategies and dealing with stress and emotional distress.

Individual therapy

Individual therapy is a therapeutic form in which a client works in direct, one-to-one contact with a therapist. This type of treatment offers a unique and intensified way to deal with mental disorders, emotional distress and personal difficulties in a safe and confidential setting.

During a one-on-one therapy session, the therapist directs his or her undivided attention to the client. The central goal is to build a trusting therapeutic relationship that allows the client to talk openly about their thoughts, feelings and behaviors. This therapeutic relationship is central to the success of the therapy, as it creates a space for honest and deep self-exploration.

Therapy usually begins with a medical history, during which the therapist collects detailed information about the client's life history, current problems, and specific symptoms. A treatment plan is then drawn up that is tailored to the individual needs and goals of the client.

Various therapeutic approaches are used in individual therapy, including cognitive behavioral therapy (CBT), psychodynamic therapy, humanistic therapy, and many others. The approach chosen depends on the therapist's training, the nature of the problems, and the client's preferences.

A significant advantage of individual therapy is the opportunity to dive deep into personal issues. The client can address topics that might be difficult to discuss in a group context. In addition, the individual attention of the therapist allows specific techniques and interventions to be used in a targeted manner and continuously adapted.

The duration of individual therapy varies greatly and depends on the type of problem being treated, individual progress, and agreed goals. It can last from a few sessions to several months or even years.

The sessions not only provide a framework for coping with current problems, but also serve personal development and the achievement of a deeper understanding of one's own self. Progress is reviewed regularly, and the treatment plan is modified accordingly to ensure that therapy remains effective.

In addition to therapeutic conversations, exercises and homework can be part of individual therapy to promote the transfer of knowledge into everyday life. This methodology helps the client to continue working on himself outside of the sessions and to consolidate changes in the long term.

Individual therapy is particularly beneficial for people who need a high degree of individual support or have specific problems that cannot be adequately addressed in a group setting. It is excellent for treating anxiety disorders, depression, trauma, relationship difficulties and many other psychological and emotional challenges.

Inner child

The concept of the "inner child" originated in humanistic and transpersonal psychology and over the years has become a central part of various psychotherapeutic approaches, including Gestalt therapy and transactional analysis. It is a metaphorical representation of the childlike aspects in each individual. These childlike parts contain all the feelings, needs, memories and experiences that were collected during childhood and unconsciously influence our behavior and thought patterns in adulthood.

The "Inner Child" can be divided into different facets in order to better understand the complexity of childhood experiences. These include, but are not limited to, the injured child, the playful child, the lonely child, and the creative child. Each of these facets represents different emotional states, needs and reaction patterns that have developed in the course of child development.

The injured child, for example, stands for experienced trauma, neglect or emotional pain, while the playful child symbolizes joy, the urge to discover and creativity. By working with the Inner Child in therapy, the aim is to find access to these deeply hidden aspects of the self. This allows the client to heal old wounds, recognize and fulfill unmet needs, as well as break through harmful patterns of behavior.

In the therapeutic context, the idea is often used that every person carries several "inner children" within them, which have stopped at different stages of development in their own history. These inner children are often responsible for recurring difficulties in relationships, emotional instability, or inexplicable patterns of behavior. Communication with the Inner Child requires careful and empathetic work, as it is often difficult to bring repressed or painful memories to the surface.

The therapeutic techniques for working with the Inner Child can be diverse and include imaginative exercises, dialogical processes, creative design and the development of care strategies for the Inner Child. Through these methods, the client is helped to create a safe inner environment in which the Inner Child is heard, seen and accepted. This not only promotes healing and integration, but also stronger inner stability and a healthy emotional experience in adulthood.

Inpatient therapy

Inpatient therapy is an intensive form of psychotherapeutic treatment in which patients remain in a specialized clinic or psychiatric facility for a certain period of time. This type of therapy is usually used when outpatient or day-care treatment measures are not sufficient to cope with the severity of the mental illness.

Inpatient therapy offers a structured daily routine and close-knit therapeutic care. The comprehensive treatment approach takes into account different therapeutic methods and disciplines such as psychotherapy, psychopharmacology, occupational therapy, art therapy, sports therapy and socio-educational support. The aim is to achieve psychological stabilisation and an improvement in patients' quality of life by combining these different approaches.

During their stay in an inpatient facility, patients receive regular individual and group therapy sessions. Individual therapies enable the therapist to specifically address individual psychological complaints and to develop tailor-made intervention strategies. Group therapies, on the other hand, promote exchange with other sufferers and the feeling of belonging, which can often have a relieving and supportive effect.

In addition, medical and nursing professionals are often available around the clock to intervene immediately if necessary. This is especially important in crisis situations or acute deterioration of mental state. Inpatient therapy thus offers a safe environment and intensive care, which are often necessary to make progress in treatment and prevent setbacks.

Another advantage of inpatient therapy is the possibility of providing temporary relief by removing it from the familiar environment and potentially stressful life situations. This can promote the recovery process and allow sufferers to fully focus on therapy without being distracted by everyday demands and stressors.

The end of inpatient therapy includes planning aftercare to facilitate the transition to everyday life and avoid relapses. This can include referral to outpatient therapists, participation in self-help groups or the use of other support services.

The duration of inpatient therapy varies greatly and depends on the severity of the disease, the individual therapy progress and the respective health insurance regulations. As a rule, the duration of treatment ranges from several weeks to a few months.

Insomnia/hyposomnia

Insomnia, also known as hyposomnia, the state of decreased sleep, are common sleep disorders that can have a profound impact on a person's mental and physical well-being. Both terms refer to difficulties in sleep behavior, but manifest themselves in different ways.

Insomnia refers to a persistent difficulty in falling asleep or staying asleep or poor sleep quality despite sufficient opportunity to sleep. Those affected often report multiple nightly waking phases, early morning awakenings without the possibility of falling asleep again, or restless sleep in general. The consequences of this disorder are far-reaching and affect various areas of life. It can lead to daytime sleepiness, exhaustion, concentration problems, irritability and reduced performance. Chronic insomnia is particularly problematic because it significantly increases the risk of mental illnesses such as depression or anxiety disorders.

Hyposomnia is a subcategory of insomnia and describes a quantitatively reduced amount of sleep. People with hyposomnia sleep fewer hours than are necessary for their health, often as a result of stress-related factors, irregular sleeping habits, or certain lifestyles. Although this reduced sleep duration can occur occasionally and be tolerated in the short term, it carries similar risks to insomnia if it is chronic. The long-term consequences include weakened immune functions, increased emotional lability and increased risk of accidents.

An accurate diagnosis by a psychotherapist or sleep specialist requires a comprehensive medical history and possibly a polysomnographic examination to rule out other medical causes. A differentiated survey is important in order to determine the exact nature and severity of the sleep disorder and to be able to develop appropriate treatment strategies.

Treatment options for insomnia and hyposomnia are diverse and range from cognitive behavioral therapy for insomnia (CBT-I) to sleep hygiene measures and drug approaches. Cognitive behavioral therapy is considered the first place to start, as it teaches specific techniques for restructuring dysfunctional thought and behavior patterns related to sleep. In addition, relaxation methods such as progressive muscle relaxation or breathing exercises can be helpful to improve the quality of sleep in the long term.

In psychotherapy, it is essential to develop therapy plans that are individually tailored to the patient, taking into account both potential causes and personal life circumstances.

Intellectual disability/oligophrenia

Intellectual disability, also known as oligophrenia, is a profound developmental disorder characterized by significantly below-average overall intellectual functioning, which is usually associated with impairments in adaptive functioning. This means that people with intellectual disabilities have difficulty developing the skills necessary in daily life, including self-care, social interaction, academic performance, and job skills.

Classification and severity

Intellectual disability is commonly classified by intelligence quotient (IQ), although this is only one aspect of a broader diagnostic process. The degrees of severity are typically divided into mild, moderate, severe and most severe intellectual disability:

- **Mild intellectual disability (IQ 50-69):** Those affected often show delayed language and motor skills, but can achieve a certain degree of independence in many everyday activities. They can often handle simple academic tasks and perform light professional activities.
- **Moderate intellectual disability (IQ 35-49):** These people need more support in coping with everyday life. You will learn basic communication skills and be

able to perform simple, routine work tasks under supervision.
- **Severe intellectual disability (IQ 20-34):** Those affected have limited language and motor skills and need ongoing support in almost all areas of daily life. Their ability to take care of themselves is severely limited.
- **Severe intellectual disability (IQ below 20):** People in this category require intensive support and care throughout. Communication is severely limited, if there is any at all, and motor skills show serious deficits.

Causes

The causes of intellectual disability are diverse and can be genetic, environmental or unknown. Genetic causes include chromosomal abnormalities such as Down syndrome, fragile X syndrome and metabolic disorders. Prenatal influences such as infections (e.g., rubella), drug and alcohol abuse during pregnancy, and complications during childbirth also play a role. Postnatal factors such as premature birth, head injuries, severe malnutrition, and conditions such as meningitis can also contribute to the development of intellectual disability.

Diagnostics

Diagnostics include a comprehensive evaluation by multidisciplinary teams, usually consisting of psychologists, pediatricians, neurologists and specialized therapists. A diagnostic approach includes the assessment of cognitive function through intelligence diagnostic tests, adaptive behavioral skills, and a thorough medical history that includes genetic, medical, and developmental information.

Therapy and support

Although intellectual disability is generally considered permanent, targeted support and therapy measures can help to maximise the potential of those affected and improve their quality of life. Early intervention programmes, specialised educational programmes, behavioural therapy interventions and the support of interdisciplinary teams are important to promote the individual skills and self-esteem of those affected.

Social implications and integration

The social integration and acceptance of people with intellectual disabilities is essential for their emotional well-being and social participation. Supportive measures, such as integration projects, inclusive learning and assisted living, help to break down prejudices and promote an inclusive society in which people with intellectual disabilities can lead an equal life.

Interpersonal Therapy (IPT)

Interpersonal Therapy (IPT) is an evidence-based, time-limited psychotherapy method that focuses on interpersonal relationships and their impact on mental health. Originally developed in the 1970s by Gerald Klerman and Myrna Weissman, it is primarily used to treat mood disorders such as depression.

IPT is based on the assumption that interpersonal relationships and social support networks play a central role in the development and maintenance of mental disorders.

The therapy focuses on current interpersonal problem areas, such as:

1. **Grieving:** The loss of an important person can cause significant depressive symptoms. IPT helps those affected to go through the grieving process and develop a new, healthy relationship with the deceased person. Adaptive coping mechanisms are promoted when changing roles and identities after the loss.
2. **Interpersonal conflicts:** Conflicts in close relationships, such as in the partnership or family, can cause considerable stress and exacerbate depressive episodes. IPT aims to identify maladaptive behaviors and communication patterns that lead to conflict and replace them with healthier alternatives.
3. **Change of role:** Life changes such as the transition from the role of employed person to retirement, the change to parenthood or leaving the parental home can cause insecurities and psychological stress. IPT supports those affected in coping with these transitions by developing adaptive adaptation strategies.
4. **Interpersonal deficits:** People who have difficulty building and maintaining stable relationships often suffer from chronic depression. IPT helps to improve social skills and learn new ways of dealing with interaction partners in order to strengthen the social network.

A characteristic feature of IPT is its structure. It is limited in time, usually to 12 to 16 sessions, and divided into different phases:

- **Initial phase:** The first sessions are characterized by the clarification of symptoms, diagnosis and identification of interpersonal problem areas. The therapist works with the patient to create a therapy formulation that provides a clear objective and structure for further treatment.
- **Middle phase:** This phase focuses on working on the identified problem areas. Specific techniques are used, such as role-plays, communication exercises, and problem-solving strategies, to bring about change in interpersonal relationships.
- **Final phase:** In the final sessions, the focus is on reviewing the therapy, recording what has been achieved and planning future strategies to cope with potential relapses. Finally, it is worked out together how the patient can continue to apply the learned skills independently.

The effectiveness of IPT has been proven by numerous studies and it has proven to be very effective, especially in the treatment of major depressive disorder. Depending on the therapy goal, IPT can also be adapted to other disorders such as eating disorders or bipolar disorder. Through its structured and targeted approach, interpersonal therapy offers a valuable and effective method for the treatment of interpersonal psychological stress.

Intervention

An intervention in psychotherapy refers to targeted and deliberate measures or interventions that the therapist carries out in order to influence the therapeutic process and advance the treatment. These measures are used systematically and methodically to direct either the patient's behavior, feelings, or thoughts in a positive direction. Basically, an intervention serves to initiate change, break patterns or open up new perspectives.

The term "intervention" encompasses a wide range of techniques and methods that can vary depending on the theoretical orientation of the therapy. In cognitive behavioral therapy (CBT), for example, an intervention can be the uncovering and changing of dysfunctional thought patterns. Here, the therapist can use techniques such as cognitive restructuring, in which the patient learns to recognize negative or distorted thoughts and replace them with more realistic and positive thought patterns.

In psychodynamic therapy, on the other hand, interventions can include depth psychological techniques such as free association or the analysis of transference and countertransference phenomena. These serve to bring unconscious conflicts and derived patterns of behavior to light.

Systemic therapy interventions, in turn, can aim to change interaction patterns within a family system. Here, for example, the therapist can use techniques such as the genogram to visually represent and analyze family structures and dynamics. Furthermore, circular questioning techniques can be used that aim to promote a change of perspective and to gain new perspectives on entrenched problems.

An intervention can be both verbal and non-verbal. Verbal interventions include questions, instructions or hints that are intended to encourage the patient to reflect or change perspective. Non-verbal interventions can have a supporting or consolidating function through posture, facial expressions and gestures.

When selecting and applying interventions, timing and the ability to fit the individual situation of the patient are decisive. The therapist must carefully consider when and what type of intervention is most effective. An intervention that is too early or inappropriate can provoke resistance or disrupt the therapeutic process.

In the ongoing dialogue between therapist and patient, the intervention is a dynamic tool that can be flexibly adapted. The patient's reactions to the intervention provide valuable feedback on its effectiveness and allow the therapist to plan the next step.

Logorrhea

Logorrhea, also known as verbal diarrhea or logomania, describes a pathologically increased talkativeness in which a person speaks uncontrollably and excessively. This phenomenon often occurs in the context of various mental disorders, primarily during manic episodes in bipolar disorder, but can also be observed in other mental states, such as schizophrenia or certain personality disorders.

People who suffer from logorrhea usually have little control over their flow of speech and often appear dominant and unstoppable in conversations. This condition often causes them to abruptly switch topics without making a logical connection to the previous content, making communicating with them challenging for others. The speed and volume of their speech may be increased, further affecting intelligibility.

In a therapeutic context, logorrhea is particularly important because it can not only indicate a diagnostic problem, but also influence the therapeutic process. A person's incessant speech can make it difficult for the therapist to make important therapeutic interventions or clarifications. Likewise, logorrhea can impair the ability of the affected person to respond appropriately to therapeutic questions or to gain reflected insights into their own situation.

It is often necessary to use specific techniques to work effectively with logorrheic patients. This includes structured conversational techniques, setting clear rules of conversation, and sometimes using medication to treat the underlying disorder. A mindful and patient attitude on the part of the therapist is crucial to support the affected person in regulating their excessive flow of speech and focusing on therapeutically relevant content.

The effects of logorrhea can be far-reaching and put a lot of strain on the social, professional and personal relationships of the person affected. Friends, family, and co-workers may feel overwhelmed or neglected, which can contribute to social isolation. Therefore, it is often necessary to develop intervention strategies in the context of psychotherapeutic treatment that involve and support the social environment of the affected person.

Research into logorrhea investigates how neurobiological, genetic and environmental factors contribute to the development of this symptomatology. In particular, the neurobiological mechanisms that take place in brain regions such as the prefrontal cortex and limbic system are the focus of scientific studies in order to gain a better understanding of the underlying causes and potential treatment options.

Mania

Mania is a mental condition characterized by persistent and abnormally high energy levels, increased mood, and increased drive activity. This extreme form of euphoria often goes far beyond normal happiness and can massively affect the daily life of the affected person. It is often observed in the context of bipolar disorder, but it can also occur in isolation or be triggered by the use of certain drugs or medications.

Typical characteristics of a manic episode are exaggerated self-esteem or ideas of size, reduced need for sleep, increased talkativeness and compulsive need to talk. In this phase, those affected tend to engage in impulsive behavior that has little regard for long-term consequences. This can manifest itself in risky decisions, such as irresponsible financial spending, promiscuous behavior, or dangerous driving.

Cognitive function and judgment are often impaired in a manic episode. People can tackle a variety of plans and projects without ultimately completing them. The train of thought is often erratic, and they skip from one topic to the next, making it hard to follow a conversation or argue coherently.

Emotions in a manic phase are intense and changeable. Although the prevailing mood is euphoric, irritability and hostility can also occur with minor frustrations or disagreement. This mood instability also contributes to social isolation, as the behavior can be difficult for those around them to understand and bear.

Severe manias can also include psychotic symptoms, such as hallucinations or delusions. This can lead to delusions of grandeur if the affected person believes that he or she is particularly talented or influential. These psychotic symptoms require immediate medical intervention because they significantly increase the risk to yourself or others.

Treatment of mania often involves a combination of drug therapy and psychotherapeutic approaches. Medications such as mood stabilizers or antipsychotics can effectively help control symptoms. Psychotherapeutic methods, especially cognitive behavioral therapy, aim to improve coping behavior and train self-awareness.

It is essential to recognize and treat a manic episode as early as possible in order to minimize long-term negative consequences. Understanding triggers and early warning signs helps both those affected and their relatives to take appropriate measures in good time and restore stability in everyday life.

Mourning

Grief is a complex and multi-layered emotional experience that occurs in response to the loss of a significant person, animal, status, ability, or other cherished connection. It is a natural and often inevitable part of human experiences and can encompass a variety of emotional, cognitive, physical, social, and behavioral responses.

Emotionally, grief often manifests itself in feelings of deep pain, overwhelming sadness, longing, loneliness, and sometimes in the form of anger or guilt. These emotions can occur in waves and vary greatly in intensity and duration. Some people experience them directly and intensely, while others may experience them with a delay or initially be less pronounced.

Cognitively, grief can influence thinking and perception. Those affected may tend to ponder the loss and its significance, which often leads to difficulty concentrating and forgetfulness. Thoughts of the deceased person or what has been lost often come to mind involuntarily. Those affected may question basic assumptions about life and their own identity, which can lead to existential considerations and a changed view of the world.

Physical symptoms are also common. These include exhaustion, sleep disorders, changes in appetite, physical complaints such as headaches or chest pain, and a general decrease in physical energy. These physical reactions are an expression of the profound psychological stress that grief entails.

Socially, grief often changes the interactions and relationships of a person affected. People in grief can withdraw, appear distant in social contacts or seek more support and closeness. The social environment plays an important role in the grieving process by providing space for the expression and exchange of feelings or by relieving the burden on the affected person through practical help.

Grief is also reflected in behavior. It can manifest itself in the form of crying, withdrawal, changing everyday routines, or activities that serve as coping strategies, such as creating rituals to remember the deceased person.

In psychotherapy, grief is recognized as an important process that requires time and space. Grief work aims to help those affected to organize their feelings, accept the loss, and eventually develop a new relationship with what has been lost. This allows them to continue on their path in life while integrating the memories of the loss into their further lives. Understanding and accompanying grief are fundamental components of therapeutic work, as each person grieves individually and has different needs and coping mechanisms.

Mutism

Mutism is a complex mental disorder that manifests itself through prolonged silence in social situations where speech is expected, even though the affected person has the language skills. This disorder is not so much an inability to speak as an inability to speak in certain contexts, often associated with significant emotional and psychological distress.

Mutism usually occurs in childhood and is often discovered at school, where children fall silent at home in a school environment despite having normal or above-average language skills. It is not a matter of simple shyness or deliberate silence, but of a complex fear reaction. This can significantly affect children's everyday social and school life and often leads to misunderstandings and social isolation.

There are different forms of mutism. Selective mutism, for example, describes silence in certain situations or in front of certain people, while the child speaks completely normally in familiar environments. Total mutism describes a situation in which the affected person does not speak at all, even in familiar surroundings and with close caregivers.

The causes of mutism are manifold. They can be genetic or caused by traumatic experiences, family conflicts and other emotional stresses. Often, deeper anxiety disorders are also the cause. A previous drastic change in the living environment, such as a move, can also act as a trigger.

The treatment of mutism requires a multidisciplinary approach. Psychotherapeutic interventions play a central role in this. Behavioral therapy is a frequently used method in which the child is systematically introduced to speaking in the fearful situations. Relaxation exercises and hypnotherapy can also be helpful in reducing underlying fears.

Cooperation with family, teachers and other caregivers also plays an important role. They should be informed and trained about the disorder so that they can act adequately and supportively. The goal is to create an anxiety-reducing environment that encourages the affected person to express themselves verbally.

It is essential to continuously monitor progress and adjust treatment accordingly. Some children need intensive therapy and long-lasting support, while others progress faster. The understanding that mutism is not a conscious decision of the affected person, but a mental disorder influenced by complex emotional and psychological factors, is elementary for successful treatment.

Narcissistic personality disorder

Narcissistic personality disorder (NPS) is a profound self-esteem disorder that usually begins in early adulthood and manifests itself in different contexts. People with this disorder show an exaggerated need for recognition and admiration, often associated with a lack of empathy for others.

A core element of NPS is a grandiose self-image. Those affected often have an inflated sense of their own importance and overestimate their abilities and achievements. They believe they are unique and special and expect to be understood or appreciated only by equally unique or high-ranking people. This self-image leads them to seek and expect recognition and admiration to an exaggerated degree.

People with narcissistic personality disorder often have difficulty tolerating criticism and react to it with anger or ignorance. Their interpersonal relationships are often marked by an imbalance, as they tend to manipulate or take advantage of other people to meet their own needs for admiration and validation. They tend to view social interactions as an opportunity to elevate their status or affirm self-evaluation.

Another central characteristic is the lack of empathy. People with NPS have difficulty empathizing with other people's feelings and needs. This can lead to interpersonal problems, as they are often perceived as inconsiderate or callous. They show little willingness to consider the perspectives of others and can sometimes react coldly or indifferently to the emotions and needs of others.

As a rule, people with this disorder possess a sensitive self-esteem that can be easily injured despite their outward grandiosity. Feedback or perceived rejection that challenges their idealized self-worth can trigger intense shame or humiliation, sometimes followed by anger or feelings of revenge.

The causes of narcissistic personality disorder are complex and diverse. A combination of genetic, biological, developmental and social factors are thought to contribute to the development of the disorder. Negative early childhood experiences, such as excessive indulgence or neglect, may also play a role.

The treatment of narcissistic personality disorder is challenging, as those affected rarely feel the need to change or gain insight into the problems of their behavior. Psychotherapeutic interventions such as cognitive behavioral therapy and psychoanalytically oriented therapy can help address underlying self-esteem issues and develop new, healthier behaviors. The inclusion of empathy and the gradual development of a realistic self-perception are central goals of the treatment.

Negative symptoms

Negative symptoms refer to the concept in clinical psychology and psychiatry that describes those symptoms in which certain abilities or behaviors have been reduced or lost. These symptoms are called "negative" because they represent a deficit or lack of normal functioning, as opposed to "positive" symptoms, which represent abnormal or excess behaviors.

A central area in which negative symptoms are particularly relevant is schizophrenia. Here it manifests itself in the form of five core aspects: affective flattening, alogy, anhedonia, avolition and social withdrawal.

Affective flattening describes a decreased emotional expressiveness and intensity. Patients often appear emotionless or show little response to emotional stimuli, which can lead to misunderstandings and social withdrawal.

Alogie refers to the impoverishment of language. Those affected have difficulty expressing themselves in detail and spontaneously and often only respond with short, monosyllabic sentences. This can affect both linguistic production and language content.

Anhedonia describes the loss of the ability to feel pleasure or pleasure in normally pleasurable activities. This can lead to reduced participation in social and leisure activities and severely affect general well-being.

Avolition refers to the reduced ability to initiate and maintain targeted activities. Sufferers often show a lack of interest or motivation to perform everyday tasks, which can lead to problems in their professional and private lives.

Social withdrawal is often a consequence of the above-mentioned deficits. The reduced ability to maintain social ties or make new contacts results in an increasing sense of isolation and an exacerbation of disease symptoms.

The treatment of negative symptoms is a major challenge, as these symptoms are often more resistant to pharmacological and therapeutic interventions than positive symptoms. Therapeutic approaches could increasingly focus on psychoeducational programs, social skills training, and individualized psychotherapies to improve the quality of life of those affected and strengthen their social skills.

The importance of negative symptoms is often underestimated in clinical practice, although it has a major influence on the quality of life and functional level of those affected. Understanding and adequately treating these symptoms requires a comprehensive and sensitive approach that takes into account both medical and psychosocial aspects.

Neologisms

Neologisms are new, often unconventional or unusual neologisms. In psychotherapy, they occur mainly in the work with clients who suffer from certain mental disorders, especially schizophrenia. These newly created words and phrases may seem meaningless or incomprehensible at first glance, but they often have a specific, personal meaning for the person concerned.

Neologisms can arise in different ways. Sometimes sufferers combine words into new entities, such as "blood black" for a particularly dark emotional experience. In other cases, completely new words can be created that do not exist in the standard language. These new formations are often characteristic of individual experiences and thought patterns of the affected persons and reflect their inner world.

For the therapist, neologisms offer valuable insights into a client's cognitive and emotional landscape. They can provide information on underlying thinking disorders, topics and conflicts that are relevant to therapeutic work. For example, a neologism formed from fear and aggression could indicate deep-rooted emotional conflicts that can be worked through in the therapeutic process.

Interpreting and working with neologisms requires a high level of sensitivity and a non-judgmental, curious attitude. It is important to understand the meaning of the neologisms in the context of the client's individual world of experience. This can be done through targeted questions and reflections within the therapeutic sessions.

In therapy, it is often helpful not to immediately correct or pathologize neologisms, but to accept them as a legitimate expression of inner states. This promotes a sense of understanding and security in the therapeutic space and can strengthen the therapeutic alliance. Sometimes a creative examination of these neologisms is also beneficial, for example through artistic or narrative techniques that encourage the client to explore and express his inner world.

Neuroasthenia (also known as fatigue syndrome)

Neuroasthenia, often referred to as fatigue syndrome, is a mental disorder that manifests itself through persistent and intense fatigue, general exhaustion, and a variety of physical and emotional symptoms. The term dates back to the 19th century and was originally introduced by George Miller Beard to describe a certain manifestation of nervous weakness that can be traced back to the so-called "modern way of life".

People affected by neuroasthenia often report persistent fatigue, even after getting enough sleep. This fatigue is often accompanied by a significant decrease in physical and mental performance, which severely affects the affected individuals. During the day, they often feel powerless and heavy, as if their energy level remains permanently at a very low level.

Other typical symptoms include difficulty concentrating, headaches, sleep disorders and increased irritability. There may be muscle tension or pain in different parts of the body. At the same time, many sufferers experience increased sensitivity to stressors and quickly feel overwhelmed or overworked. This hypersensitivity can make even mundane tasks seem insurmountable.

On an emotional level, people with neuroasthenia often struggle with anxiety, a depressed mood, and a general listlessness. A kind of inner emptiness or the feeling of being "burned out" occurs. This can become particularly problematic if people withdraw from social interactions, which can increase isolation and feelings of loneliness.

The causes of neuroasthenia are usually multifactorial. Persistent stress, overwork, insufficient recovery periods and other stresses often play a central role. Physical illnesses such as thyroid disorders or chronic infections can also contribute to the development of fatigue syndrome. In addition, there are indications that genetic factors and individual personality structures may be involved in the development of the disorder.

In psychotherapeutic practice, it is important to choose a comprehensive treatment approach that takes into account both physical and psychological aspects. A combination of psychotherapeutic interventions aimed at stress management and improving self-care and medical interventions is usually recommended. This includes relaxation techniques, cognitive behavioral therapy, and, if necessary, drug treatment to alleviate specific symptoms.

An essential part of therapy is to help those affected to develop a sense of their own limits and to learn healthy strategies for coping with stress. This often involves a restructuring of lifestyle to find a better balance between work, leisure and recreation.

Neuroplasticity

Neuroplasticity refers to the brain's ability to change its structure and function over the course of life. This ability to change allows the brain to respond to a variety of influences and experiences. It does this by creating and strengthening new neural connections, as well as weakening or eliminating existing connections.

The neurobiological basis of neuroplasticity lies in synapses, the small connections between neurons. Synaptic plasticity allows these connections to vary in strength and number. This results from various processes such as Long-Term Potentiation (LTP) and Long-Term Depression (LTD), each of which increases or decreases the efficiency of synaptic transmission.

Neuroplasticity is especially important in managing brain damage. After a stroke or traumatic brain injury, the brain can find new ways to compensate for lost functions through rehabilitation measures. This means that through targeted, repeated training, certain brain regions can be activated and strengthened, allowing them to take over functions that were previously performed by the damaged areas.

Neuroplasticity also plays an essential role in the context of psychotherapy. Many psychotherapeutic approaches, such as cognitive behavioral therapy (CBT) or mindfulness-based stress reduction (MBSR), aim to bring about changes in the brain through targeted exercises and interventions that can lead to a long-term improvement in psychological well-being. This can manifest itself in a restructuring of negative thought patterns, the reduction of anxiety symptoms or improved emotion regulation.

Learning and memory processes are also examples of neuroplasticity in everyday life. Acquiring new skills or understanding complex issues requires the effort and modification of neural networks. This is supported by constant repetition and application of what has been learned.

However, neuroplasticity is not limited to positive changes. Maladaptive patterns can also develop, for example in addictive behavior or chronic stress. In this case, the brain can be restructured in such a way that these negative behaviors or states are reinforced and maintained. Therefore, it is equally important to recognize negative plasticity and develop strategies to address and transform it.

Although neuroplasticity decreases over the course of life, it persists throughout life. This means that neuronal changes and adaptations are possible even in old age, albeit to a lesser extent. Continuous mental and physical activity goes a long way in maintaining brain plasticity.

Neurosis

Neurosis is a psychological term that describes a group of mental disorders characterized by a chronic disposition to irrational fears and emotional conflicts. Unlike psychosis, the awareness of reality remains largely intact, and the affected person is able to distinguish between his internal psychological states and the external reality.

Neuroses can manifest themselves in a variety of ways, including anxiety disorders, obsessive-compulsive disorder, hysteria, and phobic disorders. The symptoms are often distressing and affect the quality of life, but unlike psychotic episodes, they remain within a framework that maintains the basic integrity of the personality and the ability to interact socially. These disorders are often caused by inner-psychic conflicts that are rooted in early childhood and are actualized in the course of life.

The development of neuroses is traditionally considered within the framework of the psychoanalytic theory developed by Sigmund Freud. Freud postulated that mental conflicts and unprocessed, often unconscious experiences from childhood lead to unconscious fears and feelings of guilt. These internal tensions manifest themselves in neurotic symptoms. For example, a person with a compulsive personality structure may be particularly susceptible to obsessive-compulsive disorder, which is characterized by rigid thought patterns and an excessive concern for order and cleanliness.

From a therapeutic point of view, working with neurotic disorders requires a thorough medical history and research into the underlying psychological conflicts. Psychodynamic forms of therapy such as psychoanalysis or depth psychology-based psychotherapy start here by bringing the unconscious conflicts into consciousness and working through them. Cognitive behavioral therapy (CBT) can also be helpful by helping patients identify and change dysfunctional thought patterns and learn adaptive coping strategies.

Modern neuroscience has also found that neurotransmitter imbalances and certain brain areas can be involved in the development of neurotic symptoms. These findings have led to the consideration of drug approaches such as the use of antidepressants or anxiolytics to alleviate symptoms and support psychotherapy.

Neurotransmitter

Neurotransmitters are endogenous chemical substances that are synthesized and released by nerve cells (neurons) to transmit signals from one neuron to another or to other target cells, such as muscle cells or glandular cells. They play a central role in brain and nervous system function and are crucial for mediating a variety of psychological and physiological processes.

Neurotransmitters are produced in the presynaptic endings of neurons and stored in vesicles. These vesicles fuse with the presynaptic membrane at an action potential and release the neurotransmitters into the synaptic cleft. The synaptic cleft is the narrow space between the presynaptic neuron and the postsynaptic target cell. Once the neurotransmitters are released, they bind to specific receptors on the membrane of the postsynaptic cell, initiating a change in membrane potential and ultimately signal transduction.

There are several classes of neurotransmitters, including:

- **Amino acids** such as glutamate and gamma-aminobutyric acid (GABA), the most common excitatory or inhibitory neurotransmitter in the central nervous system.
- **Monoamines** such as dopamine, serotonin, and norepinephrine, which play important roles in mood, reward, sleep, and many other neuropsychological processes.
- **Peptides** such as endorphins and substance P, which are often involved in the regulation of pain and reward.
- **Acetylcholine**, which is important in both the central and peripheral nervous systems and plays a key role in the transmission of nerve impulses to muscles.

A well-known example of the function of neurotransmitters is the effect of dopamine in the brain's reward system. Dopamine is active in areas such as the ventral tegmentum and the nucleus accumbens, where it provides feelings of pleasure and reward, which is essential for motivation and learning. Dysregulation in dopamine function is associated with various mental illnesses such as schizophrenia and Parkinson's disease.

Another important example is serotonin, which is involved in regulating mood, sleep, and appetite. An imbalance of serotonin has been linked to depression and anxiety disorders. Medications such as selective serotonin reuptake inhibitors (SSRIs) aim to modulate the function of serotonin in the brain to relieve depressive symptoms.

Neurotransmitters are either broken down by enzymes, reabsorbed into the presynaptic neuron, or removed by glial cells. These mechanisms ensure that signal transmission remains precise and time-limited, which is essential for the proper functioning of the nervous system.

OCD

Obsessive-compulsive disorder (OCD) is a mental illness characterized by the presence of obsessions and/or compulsions. Both components can occur together and significantly affect the everyday life of those affected.

Obsessions:

These consist of unwanted, persistent and recurring thoughts, impulses or ideas that are experienced as stressful or frightening. Those affected often realize that these thoughts are irrational, yet they do not succeed in ignoring or suppressing them. Common themes of these thoughts can include, for example, excessive concern about dirt and germs, fear of harm, aggressive or disturbing impulses, and obsessive doubts.

Compulsive actions (compulsions):

To alleviate the anxiety and tension caused by the obsessive thoughts, the affected persons use ritualized behaviors or mental actions. These compulsions are often performed as a logical consequence of obsessive thoughts, although they do not make sense from an objective point of view. Typical examples are repeated hand washing, excessive checking, ordering rituals, counting or praying. The execution of these actions usually serves to reduce the probability of a feared event or to restore a general sense of controllability.

Epidemiology and course:

Obsessive-compulsive disorder occurs worldwide and is often diagnosed in childhood or young adulthood. There is no gender prevalence; Men and women are affected equally often. If left untreated, OCD can take a chronic course, although the severity of symptoms can vary over time. Periods of improvement are possible, but symptoms tend to be recurrent and long-lasting, which can be very distressing and limiting for sufferers.

Causes:

The exact causes of obsessive-compulsive disorder are complex and multifactorial. Genetic predispositions play a role, as do neurobiological factors, especially dysfunctions in the neural circuits associated with the processing of fear and control. Environmental factors, such as traumatic experiences or stressful life events, can also contribute to development.

Diagnostics:

The diagnosis of obsessive-compulsive disorder is primarily made through clinical interviews and special diagnostic instruments. According to the criteria of the DSM-5 or ICD-10, the symptoms must cause significant suffering, be time-consuming (more than an hour per day) or significantly impair everyday functions. Differential diagnosis must exclude other mental illnesses such as generalized anxiety disorder or phobias.

Therapy:

The treatment of obsessive-compulsive disorder usually includes a combination of psychotherapy and drug therapy.

Cognitive behavioral therapy (CBT) with exposure and response management (ERP) has proven to be particularly effective. In this process, those affected are systematically confronted with the triggering situations and gradually learn to refrain from carrying out the compulsive actions. In severe cases or if the therapy does not show the desired success, the administration of selective serotonin reuptake inhibitors (SSRIs) may be considered.

Online therapy

Online therapy, also known as internet-based psychotherapy or e-therapy, is a form of psychotherapeutic treatment that is carried out through digital means of communication such as video calls, phone calls, emails or special platforms on the internet. This method has developed and established itself strongly in recent years, especially due to the COVID-19 pandemic.

The basic structure and theoretical background of online therapy are similar to those of traditional, face-to-face psychotherapeutic sessions. The main difference is the use of digital technologies to establish and maintain contact between therapists and clients. This allows therapists to overcome geographical barriers and serve a greater number of clients, especially those who live in remote or rural areas, have mobility issues, or are otherwise difficult to reach.

Various therapeutic approaches and methods can be used in online therapy, including cognitive behavioral therapy (CBT), psychodynamic therapy, systemic therapy, and more. The effective implementation of these approaches depends on both the therapist and the client being tech-savvy and comfortable using digital communication tools.

Another essential part of online therapy is data protection and confidentiality. As therapy takes place over the internet, it is crucial that highly secure and encrypted communication platforms are used to ensure that all conversations and information exchanged remain confidential. Compliance with data protection regulations according to the GDPR (General Data Protection Regulation) in Europe and other relevant legal requirements is essential.

Online therapy offers some unique advantages compared to traditional therapy. It allows for greater flexibility in scheduling appointments and can help clients attend sessions in an environment that is comfortable for them, such as their own home. This can help make the therapy experience less stressful and more accessible.

However, there are also challenges and limitations. On the one hand, the lack of physical presence and non-verbal communication (such as posture, facial expressions and gestures) can have an impact on the therapeutic relationship and the interpretation of the client's emotional state. Technical problems such as unstable internet connections or lack of technical equipment can also be obstacles.

The burden of proof of the effectiveness of online therapy has expanded with an increasing number of studies showing positive results and success comparable to traditional methods. Nevertheless, the choice of the appropriate form of therapy remains individual and should be made taking into account the preferences and needs of the individual client as well as the special circumstances of the respective therapeutic situation.

Orthorexia

Orthorexia, also known as orthorexia nervosa, refers to a pathological fixation on the consumption of healthy foods. The term was first coined in 1997 by the American physician Steven Bratman and is derived from the Greek words "orthos" (correct) and "orexis" (appetite or desire).

People who suffer from orthorexia obsessively deal with the quality and origin of their food and develop strict rules and comprehensive rituals regarding the selection, preparation and consumption of food. This fixation can lead to significant restrictions in social and professional life, as patients tend to avoid social interactions and events where they are unable to follow their food regimes. Leisure activities that are considered a potential risk to nutritional principles are also often avoided.

Orthorexia differs from other eating disorders such as anorexia nervosa and bulimia nervosa in the sense that the focus is less on the amount of food consumed or body weight, and more on the quality and purity of the food. Sufferers often assert moral or ethical values about their diet and feel a strong sense of self-righteousness and superiority over others who do not follow these strict dietary guidelines.

The typical symptoms of orthorexia include excessive and rigid thinking about "pure" or "clean" food, strict avoidance of foods that are considered unhealthy or impure, and a feeling of fear and shame when eating foods that do not meet one's strict criteria. In addition, there can be physical consequences, such as deficiency symptoms or malnutrition, as the diet of those affected is often severely restricted and important nutrients are missing.

Treatment of orthorexia usually requires a multidisciplinary approach, including psychotherapeutic interventions, nutritional counseling, and medical supervision. Cognitive behavioral therapy (CBT) has been shown to be particularly effective in breaking through people's rigid thought patterns and behaviors and helping them develop a more balanced and less anxiety-ridden relationship with their diet. Therapy often works to help patients regain a more flexible approach to food, reduce their fear of supposedly unhealthy foods, and learn to relieve the social and psychological pressures associated with their eating habits.

Orthorexia is currently not recognized as a standalone diagnosis by the DSM-5 (Diagnostic and Statistical Manual of Mental Disorders), which makes it difficult to detect and treat the disorder. Nevertheless, awareness of orthorexia has increased in recent years, and it is increasingly recognized as a serious disorder that can have a significant negative impact on the lives of those affected.

Outpatient therapy

Outpatient therapy refers to a form of psychotherapeutic treatment in which patients continuously attend sessions in a practice or therapy centre without having to spend the night in a clinic or inpatient facility. This method of treatment is particularly flexible and can take place weekly, biweekly or in another rhythm agreed with the therapist, depending on individual needs.

A wide range of psychotherapeutic approaches and techniques is often used in outpatient therapy, such as cognitive behavioral therapy, psychoanalysis, depth psychology-based therapy and systemic therapy. The choice of therapeutic approach depends on the specific problem and the needs of the patient.

A major advantage of outpatient therapy is that patients can maintain their everyday life and social obligations as far as possible. It thus remains strongly embedded in their usual life context, which enables patients to apply and test what they have learned in a therapeutic context directly in their everyday lives. This can help stabilize the success of therapy and facilitate the transfer of therapeutic advances into daily life.

The therapeutic sessions in outpatient therapy usually last about 50 minutes. At the beginning of the therapy, a thorough anamnesis is taken, in which the therapist records the patient's symptoms and life history. Based on this, an individual treatment plan is drawn up, which is regularly reviewed and adjusted if necessary. In outpatient therapy, close and constructive cooperation between therapist and patient is essential in order to formulate and achieve common therapy goals.

The possibility of involving family members or other caregivers can also be given in outpatient therapy, especially if this contributes to solving existing problems. This is particularly relevant in systemic approaches, where the social environment is considered an essential factor for the emotional stability and well-being of the patient.

Financially, outpatient therapy is often covered by statutory or private health insurance, provided that the need for treatment is proven and a corresponding application is approved. For self-payers, there is also the possibility of taking advantage of outpatient therapy, whereby the costs are determined by agreement with the therapist.

Paramnesia

Paramnesia is a term used in psychology and psychiatry to describe a group of memory disorders in which distorted or erroneous memories occur. These can occur in different forms and vary in their severity and impact on everyday life.

A common feature of paramnesia is the mixing of actual experiences with fictional or distorted content. People who suffer from paramnesia can remember events that never happened, or they can remember real events in a completely different form than they actually happened. However, they firmly believe that their memories are correct.

One of the most well-known forms of paramnesia is déjà vu, in which the affected person believes that they have already experienced a completely new situation. The phenomenon of déjà vu is widespread and often occurs without a pathological background. However, there are also more serious forms of paramnesia that can occur in the context of mental disorders or neurodegenerative diseases.

Paramnesia can often be observed in connection with amnesia, i.e. memory loss. In such cases, those affected can replace gaps in their memory with false memories. These false memories can arise spontaneously or be caused by suggestive influences from outside, e.g. by questions from the therapist or by stories told by other people.

Another form of paramnesia is the so-called "confabulation", in which those affected, often without malicious intent, tell invented stories to fill memory gaps. Confabulation is often seen in patients with Korsakoff syndrome, a neurodegenerative disease caused by severe alcohol abuse.

The diagnosis of paramnesia requires a thorough examination by a specialist or psychotherapist. This may include a detailed medical history, cognitive tests, as well as neurological examinations. The aim of diagnostics is to identify the cause of the memory disorder and to plan appropriate therapeutic measures.

Therapeutically, there are different approaches to the treatment of paramnesia. Cognitive behavioral therapy can help identify and correct the distorted memories. In the case of neurodegenerative diseases or severe mental disorders, drug therapy may also be necessary to treat the underlying problem.

Paranoid personality disorder

Paranoid personality disorder (PPS) is a deep-rooted and persistent pattern of distrust and suspicion of other people. The defining characteristic of this disorder is a consistent sense that the intentions of others are hostile, malicious, or deceitful, even if there is no solid evidence to support this. Sufferers tend to interpret the actions of others as intentionally humiliating or as a threat to their safety and well-being.

People with paranoid personality disorder are often overly suspicious and doubt the loyalty and trustworthiness of other people, including their close friends and family members. They often experience the feeling that someone wants to harm them, betray them or deceive them. This mistrust often leads to social isolation and difficulty maintaining stable and trusting relationships.

Characteristically, sufferers are hypersensitive to criticism and tend to interpret remarks or actions of others as offensive or disparaging. They may have difficulty granting forgiveness and often hold long-lasting resentment and resentment over perceived insults or abuse.

Another common trait is the tendency to view androgynous or neutral events as personally offensive or threatening. This pattern of thinking often leads to a rigid perception and interpretation of reality, ignoring elements that do not confirm their distrust and highlighting those that seem to confirm it.

Sufferers can also maintain extreme independence, as they feel that close ties could make them vulnerable. These attachment problems can lead to them rarely revealing information about themselves and taking a strong protective stance towards their privacy.

In clinical practice, the treatment of paranoid personality disorder proves to be challenging, as patients often have difficulty trusting the therapist. Therapeutic approaches must focus on creating a safe and trusting framework in which the patient can slowly learn to question their deep-rooted mistrust and develop alternative thought patterns.

Treatment may include cognitive behavioral therapy (CBT) and other psychotherapeutic approaches that aim to identify and change unhelpful thought patterns and behaviors. An effective therapy plan also takes into account the development of social skills and stress management skills.

Common comorbidities in paranoid personality disorder include depression and anxiety disorders, which also need to be treated to achieve a holistic improvement in the quality of life of the sufferer. Finally, it is important that the therapist shows patience and empathy, as building a therapeutic alliance can often be a slow and complex process.

Parasomnias

Parasomnias are a group of sleep disorders characterized by unwanted physical or verbal behaviors during sleep. These behaviors typically occur during specific stages of sleep, especially during the transition between sleep stages, as well as between wakefulness and sleep. They can occur at any stage of sleep, however, certain types are more common at certain stages of the sleep cycle.

The main forms of parasomnias can be divided into two categories: non-REM parasomnias and REM parasomnias.

Non-REM parasomnias

Non-REM parasomnias, also known as "arousal disorders", usually occur during the deep stages of sleep (N3). The most common forms include:

- **Sleepwalking (somnambulism):** This disorder is characterized by complex motor activities that occur during sleep. Affected individuals may get out of bed, walk around, and perform simple or even complex tasks without being aware of it. Typically, in the

morning, they don't remember what they did during the episodes.
- **Night terrors (Pavor nocturnus)**: This parasomnia is characterized by sudden, panicked screams or terror from deep sleep. Unlike nightmares, these are very intense states of arousal that usually occur in the first hours of sleep. Those affected are often difficult to calm down and have little or no memory of the event after waking up.
- **Confusional arousals**: This disorder involves confusion and disorientation immediately after waking up from deep sleep. Sufferers often exhibit unusual behaviors and need more time to fully awaken.

REM parasomnias

REM parasomnias occur during REM (rapid eye movement) sleep, a phase known for intense dreaming. The most common forms include:

- **REM Sleep Behavior Disorder (RBD):** This disorder is characterized by the lack of muscle paralysis that usually occurs during REM sleep. This leads to physical activities that correspond to dreams. Those affected may scream, hit, kick or perform more complex movements. Injuries to the affected person or the partner can occur.
- **Sleep paralysis**: This occurs when waking up from REM sleep and is characterized by a temporary inability to move or speak while fully conscious. Intense and frightening hallucinations (hypnagogue or hypnopompe) are often accompanied.
- **Nightmares**: Intensely frightening dreams that often disrupt sleep and cause the affected person to wake

up and remember the dream in detail. These typically take place in the second half of the night during REM sleep.

Diagnostics and treatment

The diagnosis of parasomnias usually requires a careful medical history and sometimes polysomnographic examinations (sleep studies). This allows the exact determination of sleep stages and the identification of specific behaviors.

Therapeutic approaches vary depending on the type of parasomnia. Behavioral interventions, such as maintaining stable sleep hygiene, often play an important role. In severe cases, drug treatments may be suggested, especially if there is a risk of injury or the sleep disorder severely affects the quality of life.

Perception disorder (syn.: apperception)

In psychotherapy and psychiatry, perception disorder, also known as apperception, refers to an impairment in an individual's ability to correctly interpret sensory stimuli and to process them mentally. People who suffer from a perception disorder have difficulty recognizing the meaning of external perceptions such as sounds, images, smells or tactile stimuli and reacting appropriately to them.

These disorders can manifest themselves through various symptoms. A common feature is the abnormal or delayed response to environmental stimuli. Those affected may have problems understanding or processing complex information quickly. This can prove to be a significant disadvantage in everyday situations, such as when it comes to following a conversation, following instructions or maintaining spatial orientation.

The causes of a perception disorder are manifold. It can occur as a result of neurological diseases such as dementia or strokes. It can also be observed in the context of mental disorders such as schizophrenia or in severe depressive episodes. In addition, there are possible organic reasons, such as brain tumors, traumatic brain injuries or metabolic disorders.

The diagnosis of a perception disorder is usually made by neuropsychological tests, which are specifically aimed at analyzing cognitive functions and evaluating the ability to process information. In addition, imaging techniques such as MRI or CT can provide information about whether there are structural brain changes that could explain the disorder.

Therapeutically, treatment focuses on the underlying cause of the perception disorder. If a neurological disease is present, drug and rehabilitative therapy may be necessary. In the case of mental disorders, psychotherapeutic interventions, possibly combined with drug treatment, are in the foreground. A multidisciplinary approach involving neurologists, psychiatrists, psychotherapists and occupational therapists can be particularly effective here.

Furthermore, it can be helpful to carry out specific training sessions to improve cognitive function. These trainings can include exercises aimed at increasing attention and concentration skills and improving sensory integration.

Family members and caregivers should be educated about the nature and limitations of the disorder of perception in order to create a supportive and understanding environment that can help improve the quality of life of the person affected.

Personal history

The patient's own medical history describes the process in which the patient independently collects information about his or her own medical history and current complaints and makes it available to the treating therapist. This includes not only the collection of facts about previous mental and physical illnesses, but also the subjective assessment of symptoms, experiences and experiences that the patient considers relevant.

The self-anamnesis often begins before the first therapy session and can be done by means of standardized questionnaires or freely designed reports. The patient has the opportunity to reflect on his symptoms and to find an initial approach to his or her own problems. Specific symptoms as well as emotional, cognitive and behavioral aspects can play a role.

A significant advantage of the self-anamnesis is the promotion of self-reflection and self-perception. The patient is encouraged to think about his inner states and external experiences, which can already be therapeutically effective. In addition, the independent development of the anamnesis helps the patient to take an active role in the therapeutic process.

In the therapeutic practice, the patient's own anamnesis is discussed and supplemented at the beginning of the therapy sessions. The therapist can ask specific questions to clear up ambiguities or to further deepen specific topics. This enables a holistic view of the patient's problems and helps to develop an individual and tailor-made treatment concept.

The self-anamnesis not only provides useful information for diagnosis, but also lays the foundation for a trusting therapeutic relationship. The patient feels taken seriously and actively involved in the process. This can lead to better compliance and a more constructive working alliance between patient and therapist.

Another aspect of the patient's own anamnesis is the recording of the patient's resources and strengths. By looking back at their past and present, the patient can identify their own coping strategies and success factors that may be useful for the therapeutic process.

Personality disorder

A personality disorder is a mental health problem characterized by deep-rooted, long-term patterns of behavior and inner experiences that deviate significantly from the expectations of the individual's culture. These patterns are inflexible, pervasive, and begin during adolescence or early adulthood.

People with personality disorders often experience severe difficulties in their relationships and in their professional or social environment. Their thoughts, feelings, and behaviors are dysfunctional in many situations and often lead to conflict or difficulty interacting with others. Those affected often cannot recognize that their perceptions and behaviors are inappropriate or problematic, which makes treatment difficult.

There are several types of personality disorders, which are divided into clusters:

1. **Cluster A: Strange and eccentric disorders:**
    - **Paranoid personality disorder**: Characterized by distrust and suspicion of others, which causes the motives of others to be interpreted as malicious.
    - **Schizoid personality disorder**: Excessive emotional detachment and limited expression in interpersonal relationships.
    - **Schizotypal personality disorder**: Social and interpersonal deficits characterized by acute discomfort in close relationships and bizarre thoughts or behaviors.

2. **Cluster B: Dramatic, emotional and erratic disorders:**
    - **Antisocial personality disorder**: A pattern of disregard and violation of the rights of others, lack of social responsibility, and repeated violations of the law.
    - **Borderline personality disorder**: Intense and unstable interpersonal relationships, extreme black-and-white thinking, unstable self-image, and intense emotional reactions.
    - **Histrionic personality disorder**: Excessive emotionality and a strong need for attention, as well as dramatic and theatrical behaviors.

- **Narcissistic personality disorder**: A grandiose self-image, a deep need for admiration, and a lack of empathy for others.

3. **Cluster C: Anxious and fearful disorders:**
    - **Avoidant-self-insecure personality disorder**: Extreme social inhibition, feelings of inadequacy and hypersensitivity to negative evaluation.
    - **Dependent personality disorder**: An excessive need to be cared for, leading to submissive and clingy behavior, as well as fear of separation.
    - **Obsessive-compulsive personality disorder**: A pattern of perfectionism and orderly behavior that comes at the expense of flexibility, openness, and efficiency.

Treatment for personality disorders can be complex and lengthy. It usually includes psychotherapy, using various approaches such as cognitive behavioral therapy (CBT), dialectical behavioral therapy (DBT), or psychodynamic therapy. Medications can be used if necessary, especially if there are comorbid disorders such as depression or anxiety disorders.

Phobia

A phobia is a form of anxiety disorder characterized by an excessive and irrational fear of certain objects, situations, or activities. This fear is disproportionate to the actual danger posed by the anxiety-inducing stimulus.

Phobias can be divided into three main categories: specific phobias, social phobia, and agoraphobia. Specific phobias refer to an intensified fear of a particular object or situation, such as arachnophobia (fear of spiders), claustrophobia (fear of confined spaces), or acrophobia (fear of heights). Social phobia, also known as social anxiety disorder, includes the fear of social or performance-related situations in which a person fears being judged or evaluated negatively. Finally, agoraphobia refers to the fear of places or situations where escape would be difficult or no help seems available.

People with phobias often make significant efforts to avoid the anxiety-inducing objects or situations. These avoidance strategies can significantly affect daily life and limit quality of life. Physical symptoms that can occur in phobic situations include palpitations, sweating, trembling, dizziness, and difficulty breathing. These physical reactions are an expression of the activation of the autonomic nervous system, especially the sympathetic nervous system, which triggers the fight-or-flight response.

The development of phobias is often understood as an interplay of genetic, biological, psychological and environmental factors. A genetic predisposition can make certain people more susceptible to developing anxiety disorders. Learning theories suggest that phobias can arise from classical conditioning, in which a neutral stimulus (e.g., a spider) is associated with an unpleasant event (e.g., pain), eventually leading to the development of a phobic response.

Treatment of phobias can include different approaches. One of the most effective methods is cognitive behavioral therapy (CBT), which uses techniques such as exposure therapy and cognitive restructuring. Exposure therapy helps the patient to face the anxiety-inducing stimulus gradually and in a controlled manner, while cognitive restructuring aims to identify and change dysfunctional thought patterns. In addition, medications, such as antidepressants or anxiolytics, can be used to relieve anxiety symptoms, especially if the phobia is severe.

Pica in childhood

Pica is an eating disorder characterized by the repeated eating of non-nutritive substances that are unusual for the child's age and development. In children, this often includes consuming things like soil, chalk, paper, paint, clay, dirt, or even hair. These bouts of eating non-edible objects must last at least a month to be diagnosed as pica.

Causes of pica can be varied and include both medical and psychological aspects. Medical causes include, for example, a nutrient deficiency, such as iron or zinc deficiency, which can lead to unusual cravings. Psychological causes can be associated with a developmental disorder or another mental disorder, such as autism spectrum disorders or intellectual disabilities. In some cases, emotional stress, such as neglect or a disturbed family dynamic, can also lead to pica.

The child's behavior at pica can involve risks to both physical health and psychological development. For example, any health risks may include the risk of infection, poisoning, intestinal obstruction or injury to the surface of the digestive tract. The repetitive behavior can have an impact on normal psychological and social development because it can prevent the child from other activities and social interactions.

Therapeutic approaches to pica require a multidisciplinary approach that includes both medical and psychotherapeutic interventions. Initially, a medical examination is often carried out to rule out or treat any underlying physical causes such as nutrient deficiencies or poisoning. Psychotherapeutic interventions often involve behavioral therapy, which aims to reduce the unwanted eating behavior and replace it with more appropriate behaviors. Parent training and education are also essential parts of the treatment plan to effectively engage parents in supporting and monitoring their children.

The prognosis of pica in childhood depends heavily on the underlying cause and the effectiveness of the therapeutic measures initiated. The earlier the disorder is detected and treated, the better the long-term prospects of successfully overcoming the behavior.

Pledge of secrecy

Confidentiality is a central ethical and legal principle in psychotherapy. It forms the basis for the relationship of trust between therapist and client and guarantees that all content and information discussed in therapy is neither passed on to third parties nor used outside of therapy sessions.

The origin of confidentiality can be found in medical professional ethics and is enshrined in law in most countries. Psychotherapists are therefore obliged to protect the privacy and personal data of their clients.

The duty of confidentiality includes all information that therapists learn in the course of their professional activities. This includes all the content of the conversations, data about the client's personality, his medical and psychological history, as well as diagnoses and treatment plans. Documentation and records that are created in the course of therapy are also covered by the duty of confidentiality and must be stored securely.

However, there are exceptions to this rule. For example, confidentiality can be broken in emergencies, for example if there is acute danger to oneself or others and it is necessary to pass on information to other persons or institutions in order to avert a danger. The duty of confidentiality can also be broken if the client expressly consents in writing to the disclosure of certain information. Another exceptional case is when courts or authorities require information that is required by law.

Violation of confidentiality can have serious legal and professional consequences. Criminal sanctions include fines and imprisonment, among others. Civil law consequences such as claims for damages and professional measures, up to and including the loss of the professional license, are also possible.

The importance of confidentiality cannot be overestimated in practice. It allows clients to talk openly about their most intimate thoughts, feelings, and problems without having to worry about this information being leaked to the public. Thus, confidentiality contributes significantly to the effectiveness of therapeutic work and supports the mental health and well-being of the clients.

Positive symptoms

In psychotherapy and psychiatry, the term "positive symptoms" refers to a group of conspicuous symptoms that occur in certain mental disorders, especially schizophrenia. These symptoms are called "positive" because they add something to a person's normal behavior or thinking, as opposed to "negative symptomatology," which is characterized by the absence or reduction of normal functions.

A central feature of positive symptoms are hallucinations. Hallucinations are perceptions without an external source of stimulus and can affect all sensory modalities, with auditory hallucinations (hearing voices or sounds) being the most common. Patients often report hearing voices commenting on what they are doing or giving them orders, which can cause significant stress and distress.

Another key element of positive symptoms is delusions. Delusions are fixed, false beliefs that cannot be corrected by rational argument and are often bizarre or disproportionate. Common forms of delusions are paranoia (the belief that one is being spied on or persecuted), delusions of grandeur (the belief that one possesses special power, importance, or knowledge), and relational delusions (the belief that random events or comments are related to oneself).

In addition, those affected can suffer from disorganized thinking and speaking. This is evident in the inability to speak logically and coherently; Sentences and thoughts can end abruptly or deviate in unpredictable directions. In addition, neologisms, i.e. the invention of new words or concepts, often occur that make no sense to outsiders.

Disorganized behavior is also a typical feature of positive symptoms. Sufferers can perform unpredictable or seemingly purposeless actions, ranging from a lack of purposefulness to extreme motor disorders. Examples of this are catatonia, where the level of movement is greatly reduced or bizarre postures are adopted.

Aggressive or agitated behaviors are also occasionally part of the positive symptoms. These can manifest themselves in excessive irritability and a tendency to impulsive behavior and often pose a danger to those affected themselves or to others.

Post-traumatic stress disorder (PTSD)

Post-traumatic stress disorder (PTSD) is a mental illness that occurs in response to a traumatic event. Such events can be experienced during armed conflicts, serious accidents, natural disasters, physical or sexual assaults or other threatening situations. The essence of PTSD is that the affected person has experienced the event as highly stressful and overwhelming and has not been able to process the threat experienced emotionally or cognitively.

A person with PTSD suffers from a variety of symptoms that can be divided into four main categories: reliving the trauma, avoidance and emotional numbness, changes in arousal and reactions, and negative changes in thoughts and mood.

Reliving the trauma can come in the form of recurring, intrusive memories, nightmares, and flashbacks. In these moments, the affected person relives the traumatic situation in their thoughts, as if it were taking place in the here and now. These experiences can be extremely real and frightening.

Avoidance and emotional numbness manifest themselves in the affected person's intense avoidance of situations, places, or people associated with the trauma. At the same time, a general withdrawal from interpersonal relationships and activities that previously gave pleasure can be observed. Feelings of emotional emptiness or separation from other people are also typical.

Changes in arousal and reactions are characterized by increased readiness to react and states of tension. This can include constant vigilance against potential dangers (hypervigilance), irritability and outbursts of anger, and sleep disturbances. Other symptoms in this category include difficulty concentrating and increased jumpiness at unexpected noises or events.

Negative changes in thoughts and mood can include feelings of guilt and shame, decreased self-esteem, numbness, and persistent, negative beliefs about oneself or the world. Sufferers may have difficulty feeling positive emotions and feel a sense of hopelessness about the future.

The diagnosis of PTSD is usually carried out through structured interviews and specific questionnaires aimed at recording the presence and severity of the various symptoms. An important aspect of diagnosis is that symptoms persist for more than a month and lead to significant impairment in social, occupational, or other important functional areas.

Therapeutic approaches to the treatment of PTSD include both psychotherapeutic and drug interventions. Evidence-based psychotherapeutic methods include cognitive behavioral therapy (CBT), especially trauma-focused CBT, and Eye Movement Desensitization and Reprocessing (EMDR). These therapies aim to gradually process and integrate the stressful memories and their emotional effects.

In the medical field, antidepressants are often used to alleviate the symptoms. Accompanying support from social workers, self-help groups and complementary therapy methods such as body therapy or mindfulness training can also be helpful.

Pre-suicidal syndrome

Pre-suicidal syndrome is a special constellation of psychological states and behaviors that is often observed in people who show an increased risk of suicide. This term was coined by the Austrian psychiatrist Erwin Ringel and includes three central characteristics: constriction, aggression reversal and suicidal fantasies.

1. Constriction:

The affected person experiences an increasingly limited perception of their environment and their possibilities for action. This can manifest itself on an emotional, mental and situational level. Emotionally, this means a flattening of feelings and the loss of the ability to experience joy or positive sensations. Mentally, the constriction leads to tunnel vision-like states in which thoughts constantly revolve around certain topics, usually one's own failure, feelings of guilt or hopelessness. Depending on the situation, this means that those affected are no longer able to recognize alternative solutions to their problems or accept help from outside.

2. Aggression reversal:

Aggression and destructive impulses, which could actually be directed at external persons or situations, are turned inwards against one's own person. This manifests itself in self-reproach, especially feelings of worthlessness and failure. Self-injurious behavior can also be an expression of this aggression reversal. Those affected feel a deep sense of self-depreciation and may unconsciously look for ways to punish themselves for supposed mistakes or weaknesses.

3. Suicidal fantasies:

A growing idea of the possibility of suicide as a kind of "last resort" is developing. These fantasies can vary from fleeting thoughts of death to detailed planning of suicide. The thought of ending one's own life often plays an ambivalent role: on the one hand, it can be perceived as relieving, but on the other hand, it can also cause additional fears and uncertainties.

The term pre-suicidal syndrome serves, on the one hand, to make therapists more sensitive to signs of a possible risk of suicide and, on the other hand, to take preventive measures at an early stage. The complexity and interaction of these three central characteristics clearly show that a more in-depth diagnosis and often an interdisciplinary approach are necessary to counteract suicidal and self-harm intentions.

To ensure effective intervention, it is essential to create an open, trusting climate of conversation in which the affected person feels safe to openly express their thoughts and feelings, including suicidal impulses. This enables a precise assessment of the risk and provides the basis for targeted therapeutic and possibly psychiatric support.

Professional Code of Conduct

The Professional Code of Conduct is a set of rules that defines the professional and ethical standards as well as the rights and duties of psychotherapists. It serves to ensure quality and protect patients and is issued by the respective psychotherapeutic professional associations and chambers. The Professional Code gives detailed instructions on various aspects of professional practice and deals with a wide range of topics that are important for professional practice.

One topic of the professional code is the duty of confidentiality. Psychotherapists are obliged to treat all information entrusted to them in the course of their professional activities confidentially. This regulation serves to protect the privacy of patients and is elementary for the relationship of trust between therapist and patient. Without the assurance of confidentiality, it would be difficult for many people to open up to the challenges and problems they want to address in a therapeutic context.

Another important area of the professional code concerns vocational training and further education. Psychotherapists are obliged to undergo continuous training in order to maintain and expand their professional skills. The professional code determines the extent and areas in which further education and training must be completed, thus ensuring that therapists are always up to date with the latest research and practice.

The professional code also contains regulations on the practice of the profession and the conduct of practice. These include regulations on the furnishing and equipment of practice rooms as well as on the framework conditions of therapy. Specifications are also made for the documentation of the therapeutic work. This includes both the documentation of therapy courses and outcomes and the proper storage of patient records.

Ethical principles are another important part of the professional code. These principles are intended to ensure that psychotherapists respect and promote the human dignity and autonomy of their patients in their professional activities. This includes guidelines for dealing with power and dependence in the therapeutic relationship as well as for avoiding conflicts of interest. Regulations on sexual and emotional relationships between therapists and patients also belong to this area and help to maintain professional distance and integrity.

The professional code also defines the forms and procedures for dealing with violations of professional law. These regulations include the description of the sanctions that can be imposed in the event of violations of professional duties as well as the corresponding complaint and disciplinary procedures. These mechanisms ensure that appropriate measures are taken to ensure the quality of therapeutic care and the safety of patients in the event of non-compliance with professional standards.

Professional ethics

Professional ethics in psychotherapy encompasses the moral and professional principles that therapists follow to treat their patients appropriately and respectfully. These principles serve as guidelines for responsible action and decision-making in a therapeutic context. Professional ethics forms the foundation of the relationship of trust between therapist and patient and ensures the integrity and professionalism of the therapeutic process.

A feature of professional ethics is confidentiality. Psychotherapists are obliged to protect all information entrusted to them in the course of therapy. This means that no personal data or conversation content may be passed on without the patient's explicit consent. However, in certain exceptional situations, such as danger to the life of the patient or third parties, this rule can be put into perspective.

Another principle is that of autonomy and respect for the patient's self-determination. Therapists respect the individual rights and decisions of their patients and promote their ability to make self-determined decisions. This includes education about therapeutic methods and possible risks so that patients can consent to therapy on an informed basis.

At the same time, professional ethics emphasizes the need to maintain competence. Therapists should continuously update their specialist knowledge through further education and training in order to be able to offer high-quality and up-to-date therapeutic services. This includes the willingness to seek supervision or collegial advice in complex cases.

The integrity of the therapist is another important aspect of professional ethics. Therapists should be honest and sincere in their profession and avoid any form of deception or manipulation. This applies to both the therapeutic process and administrative aspects such as the billing of services.

After all, professional ethics also include professional distance. It is imperative to avoid personal relationships with patients that could go beyond the therapeutic relationship to prevent conflicts of interest and emotional entanglements. This distance makes it possible to remain objective and impartial.

The principles of professional ethics are enshrined in various professional codes and guidelines, such as the ethical guidelines of professional associations. They serve both to protect patients and to ensure the professional standards of psychotherapy.

Professional ethics requires therapists to continuously reflect on themselves and critically question their actions in order to enable ethically impeccable, respectful and patient-centered therapy.

Professional indemnity

Professional liability insurance is an essential insurance policy for psychotherapists. It protects the therapist from the financial consequences of claims for damages that may arise from professional activity. In practice, this means that the insurance takes effect if patients or third parties suffer damage as a result of the therapist's professional activity and claim damages.

One component of professional liability insurance is protection against the usual occupational risks. If, for example, a patient claims to have suffered physical or mental damage as a result of therapy, the insurance company will cover the legal examination and the costs of any claims settlement in the event of a claim. The same applies to possible financial losses that could arise from incorrect or incorrect treatment.

In addition, professional indemnity often includes a passive legal protection function. This consists of fending off unjustified or excessive claims. So if a patient makes unjustified claims, the insurance company will cover the defense, including legal and court costs.

Another important element of professional liability insurance is the so-called risks arising from the status of employer. If a psychotherapist employs employees, there could be claims for damages resulting from the employment of the employees. Professional liability insurance also protects against financial claims in these cases.

The sum insured by the insurance is also a critical point. It determines the maximum amount up to which the insurance company will pay in the event of a claim. This should be chosen sufficiently high to be covered even in the event of major damage. Many insurance companies offer different tariffs tailored to the specific needs and risks of each practice.

In addition, there are special variants of professional liability, such as psychotherapist liability, which are tailored to the special requirements and risks in this professional field. These insurances take into account the specific characteristics of psychotherapeutic work and often offer extended services such as insurance cover in the event of violations of confidentiality.

Projection

Projection is a psychological defense mechanism in which a person unconsciously transfers their own unwanted feelings, thoughts or characteristics that they cannot accept in themselves to other people. Instead of acknowledging and integrating these negative aspects as part of their reality, they are shifted to the outside world and attributed to others. This serves the purpose of maintaining one's own self-image and avoiding emotionally stressful insights or conflicts.

The mechanism of projection can manifest itself in different ways. A common form is the projection of fear or aggression. For example, a person who secretly harbors strong hostile feelings toward someone might perceive those feelings as threatening and therefore believe that the other person has hostile intentions toward them. Perception is distorted so that one's own feelings are interpreted as reactions of others.

Another context in which projection often occurs is in the area of relationship dynamics. Within interpersonal relationships, it can happen that someone projects their own insecurities or weaknesses onto their partner. For example, someone who feels unattractive might constantly suspect that their partner has lost interest, or someone who feels guilty might accuse others of criticizing them for their behavior.

In therapeutic work, the identification and understanding of projections is an important component. Through gentle and targeted therapeutic interventions, patients can learn to recognize and withdraw their projected feelings and thoughts. This allows them to develop a more realistic view of their relationships and their environment, as well as to achieve a more integrated self-image.

A vivid example of projection is the work in the context of psychoanalysis, where Sigmund Freud coined this term and described it in detail. In therapy, various techniques can be used to help patients identify their projections. This can be done through conversations, role-plays, or the use of projective tests such as the Rorschach test. Through these methods, hidden contents of the unconscious can be brought to the surface and processed.

A deeper understanding of projection also leads to the insight that the origin of these displacements is often found in early childhood experiences. Children develop this mechanism as a form of self-protection to deal with stressful feelings and experiences. These early learned patterns often persist into adulthood if they are not made aware and replaced by new behaviors.

Working on projections not only promotes the personal growth of the individual, but also contributes to the improvement of interpersonal relationships. By learning to take responsibility for their own feelings and thoughts, individuals can counteract the mechanisms of blame and misunderstandings. In the long term, this leads to a more stable and authentic form of communication and interaction in personal and professional terms.

Psychiatric emergencies

Psychiatric emergencies are acute mental conditions that require immediate medical and therapeutic intervention to avert serious danger to the affected person or those around them. These situations can be brought on by a variety of causes, including severe mental illness, drug or alcohol use, traumatic experiences, or other psychosocial stresses.

Typical psychiatric emergencies include:

1. **Suicidal crises**: This is one of the most urgent forms of psychiatric emergencies. Patients in a suicidal crisis often show despair, hopelessness, and concrete plans or intentions to take their own lives. Immediate intervention is required to protect the patient's life and initiate intensive psychotherapeutic measures.
2. **Acute psychoses**: Patients who suffer from acute psychosis experience a loss of touch with reality. You may have hallucinations (perceptual distortions such as hearing voices) and delusions (false beliefs such as paranoia). These conditions can lead to dangerous behavior, so that rapid drug and therapeutic treatment is often necessary.
3. **Aggressive or violent behavior**: It becomes particularly threatening when patients pose a danger to themselves or others due to their mental state. This can take the form of physical violence, destructive behavior, or self-harm. A combination of de-escalation techniques and possibly pharmacological interventions is needed here.
4. **Acute stress reactions**: After extremely stressful or traumatic events, patients can develop overwhelmingly strong emotional reactions. Symptoms such as panic attacks, dissociations, or severe anxiety may occur, and there is a high risk of developing post-traumatic stress disorder (PTSD). Immediate psychological support and stabilization of the patient is crucial here.
5. **Delirium**: This condition is characterized by sudden confusion, clouding of consciousness, and cognitive impairment, often due to medical or neurological causes such as infections or drug intoxication. Rapid diagnosis and treatment of the underlying causes are

necessary to avoid potentially life-threatening complications.
6. **Substance-induced crises**: The abuse of substances such as alcohol, illegal drugs or medication can lead to acute psychological emergencies. Symptoms can range from severe withdrawal symptoms to toxic psychotic states. Detoxification and stabilization of the patient require close monitoring and support from healthcare professionals.

In the handling of psychiatric emergencies, a quick and precise assessment of the situation, adequate crisis intervention and subsequent planning of further diagnostic and therapeutic measures play a central role. The collaboration of different disciplines, including psychiatrists, psychotherapists, emergency physicians and nurses, is often essential to ensure optimal care and minimize the danger to the affected person and their environment.

Psychoanalysis

Psychoanalysis is a far-reaching theoretical and clinical concept developed by Sigmund Freud in the late 19th and early 20th centuries. It offers an insight into human behavior that is influenced by the unconscious. Freud's theory assumes that many of our thoughts, feelings, and actions are driven by unconscious drives and conflicts, which often have their roots in early childhood.

A central concept of psychoanalysis is the conflict between the three structures of the psyche: the id, the ego and the superego. The id represents the primitive, instinctual needs and desires. It acts according to the pleasure principle and seeks immediate satisfaction. The ego develops in order to mediate between the unconscious instinctual desires of the id and the demands of reality. It works according to the principle of reality. The superego develops and represents the internalized moral standards of society and parents. It acts as a kind of conscience that evaluates and, ideally, regulates the behavior of the individual.

An essential part of psychoanalytic therapy is free association, where the patient is asked to speak freely and express every thought and feeling that comes to mind, without censorship or restraint. This allows the therapist to gain insights into the patient's unconscious and uncover hidden conflicts and repressed memories.

Dream interpretation is another important aspect of psychoanalysis. Freud believed that dreams are "the royal road to the unconscious" and that they contain coded messages that can reveal the dreamer's hidden desires and fears. By analyzing dreams, the therapist can gain deeper insights into the patient's unconscious processes.

Transference and countertransference are also central concepts in psychoanalysis. Transference occurs when the patient transfers feelings that were originally felt towards important people in childhood to the therapist. This can include both positive and negative feelings and provides valuable information about the patient's relationships and conflicts. Countertransference refers to the therapist's emotional response to the patient and their transferences.

Psychoanalytic therapy can often take several years to complete, as it is a deep and comprehensive process that aims to bring about long-term changes in the patient's thinking and behavior. The aim is to help the patient gain a deeper understanding of himself, to work through his unconscious conflicts and thus to improve his psychological well-being.

Psychoanalysis has undergone many evolutions and criticisms over time, but its basic principles have exerted a significant influence on the entire psychotherapeutic landscape and remain present in many therapeutic directions.

Psychodynamic therapy

Psychodynamic therapy is a psychotherapeutic method based on depth psychology and stands in the tradition of classical psychoanalysis. Its goal is to understand and work on the unconscious psychological processes and inner conflicts that influence an individual's behavior and experience. Common areas of application are depression, anxiety disorders, personality disorders and a wide variety of psychosomatic illnesses.

At the heart of psychodynamic therapy is self-exploration. Therapist and client work closely together to explore the roots of emotional difficulties. These are often deeply rooted in childhood and manifest themselves later in life as symptoms or problematic behaviors.

A core theory of psychodynamic therapy is the model of the unconscious. Humans are seen as beings whose actions and feelings are influenced by unconscious motives and conflicts. By exploring these unconscious contents in the therapeutic setting, client and therapist can shed light on hidden desires, fears and inner conflicts together.

A central mechanism of psychodynamic therapy is transference. This refers to the phenomenon that clients transfer feelings and reaction patterns that were originally reserved for important caregivers such as parents or siblings to the therapist. The therapist uses this transmission to gain insights into the client's relationship patterns and interpersonal dynamics.

Countertransference is another essential concept. Here, the therapist reflects on his own emotional reactions to the client. These reactions can provide valuable clues to the dynamics between therapist and client and enrich the therapeutic work, provided that the therapist is aware of his or her countertransference feelings and handles them professionally.

Creativity and flexibility of the therapist are crucial for the success of the treatment. The therapist must be able to use intuitive insights and apply them to the client's specific needs. This requires a deep understanding of both theoretical concepts and the human psyche.

Fantasy and dreams are also important aspects of psychodynamic therapy. Dreams are seen as a window to the unconscious and offer important clues to inner conflicts and unconscious desires. Dream analysis makes it possible to interpret the symbolic and emotional content of dreams and to work out their relevance for the client's current experience.

The duration of the treatment is variable and can range from a few months to several years, depending on the depth of the issues to be worked on and the individual needs of the client. Nevertheless, the focus is on achieving sustainable change and deeper self-knowledge.

Psychoeducation

Psychoeducation refers to the structured and methodologically sound process of imparting knowledge and skills to patients and their relatives in the context of psychotherapeutic treatment. The aim of this knowledge transfer is to promote the understanding of mental illnesses, their causes and their treatment options and thus to have a positive influence on the course of the disease and therapy acceptance.

In psychoeducation, specific knowledge is presented in an understandable and everyday way. Various methods and media can be used, such as individual or group sessions, information materials, audiovisual media or interactive workshops. The topics of psychoeducation can be very diverse and range from basic information about the diagnosis and symptoms of an illness to strategies of self-management and crisis management.

A central component of psychoeducation is the destigmatization of mental illnesses. By educating patients and relatives about the biological, psychological and social causes of mental disorders, they can develop a deeper understanding of the disease. This often reduces the shame and guilt that can come with mental illness and encourages more open communication about the issues that exist.

Psychoeducation also aims to teach affected individuals specific skills that can be helpful in dealing with the condition. These include techniques for dealing with stress, relapse prevention, strategies for improving social interaction, and recognizing and coping with negative thought patterns. These skills help patients to improve their autonomy and quality of life and to actively participate in social life.

In practice, it has been shown that psychoeducation is often used as a supplementary measure to psychotherapeutic treatment. In cognitive behavioral therapy (CBT), for example, it is an important component in enabling patients to reflect on their disease and thus contribute to positive change on their own. In systemic therapy, too, the involvement of the family and other social networks through psychoeducation can be beneficial in order to achieve the therapeutic goal.

Ultimately, psychoeducation serves not only to impart knowledge, but also to strengthen the relationship of trust between therapist and patient. This is done through open and respectful communication, which is the basis of every successful therapeutic relationship.

Through systematic education and support, those affected are given tools to help them better cope with the challenges of everyday life and actively participate in their recovery process, which can lead to more stable mental health in the long term.

Psychosomatics

Psychosomatics is a medical and psychotherapeutic concept that examines and treats the interactions between body and psyche. The term comes from the Greek: "Psyche" means soul and "Soma" means body. Psychosomatics refers to the research and therapy of diseases in which physical symptoms are influenced or caused by psychological or emotional factors.

Psychosomatic illnesses are physical illnesses that cannot be explained by organic findings alone, but in which psychological factors play an essential role. These diseases often manifest themselves in various forms, such as chronic pain, functional complaints and somatoform disorders. Well-known examples can be stomach ulcers, irritable bowel syndrome, asthma, cardiovascular diseases and certain skin diseases.

In psychosomatics, it is assumed that the body acts as a resonating body for mental conflicts. Stress, unprocessed trauma, unresolved emotional conflicts or deep-rooted fears can manifest themselves physically. The body reacts to these mental stresses through symptoms that often have to be seen as warning signals. The focus here is on a holistic view of the person: not only the physical complaints, but also the mental and social environment of the patient are included in the diagnosis and therapy.

Diagnostically, psychosomatics makes use of both physical medical and psychological procedures. In addition to the medical examination and medical history, this also includes psychological tests and detailed discussions to identify possible psychological causes of the physical symptoms. Various approaches are used in the therapeutic area, including depth psychological therapy, behavioral therapy, systemic therapy and relaxation methods. Body-oriented forms of therapy such as physiotherapy or respiratory therapy can also be an integral part of treatment.

An important element of psychosomatics is the promotion of self-perception and self-knowledge. Patients are encouraged to recognize and understand a connection between their feelings, thoughts and physical complaints. In this way, they can learn to better cope with stress and emotional distress and improve their physical and mental health in the long term.

Psychosomatics requires close interdisciplinary cooperation between different disciplines such as general medicine, psychiatry, psychotherapy, physiotherapy and social work. This cooperation enables a comprehensive and effective treatment of patients that aims to do more than just alleviate symptoms, but to improve the quality of life holistically.

By acknowledging the complex interactions between the body and the psyche, psychosomatics offers a valuable integrative approach to promoting and maintaining health.

Psychotherapy

Psychotherapy is an intensive and systematic process of treating mental disorders, emotional difficulties, and various forms of suffering that affect a person's daily life. It is based on a cooperative relationship between a psychotherapist and a client, with the aim of achieving a positive change in the client's mental state and behaviour through targeted interventions, conversations and methods.

Psychotherapy encompasses a variety of approaches and techniques based on different theoretical foundations. Among the best known are cognitive behavioral therapy, psychoanalysis, humanistic therapy, systemic therapy, and integrative therapy. Each of these approaches has its own models for explaining mental health problems and its specific methods of treating it.

Cognitive behavioral therapy (CBT), for example, aims to identify and change dysfunctional thought patterns and behaviors. Negative thoughts and beliefs are replaced by more realistic and positive perspectives, leading to an improvement in emotional well-being.

Psychoanalysis, which was founded by Sigmund Freud, focuses on the unconscious life of the soul and the role of early childhood experiences. It examines the deeply hidden conflicts and longings that can manifest themselves in symptoms and problematic behaviors.

Humanistic therapies, such as Carl Rogers' Client-Centered Therapy, emphasize the potential of humans for self-realization and the importance of an empathetic and authentic therapeutic relationship. The focus here is on promoting self-esteem and personal development.

In systemic therapy, the client is not considered in isolation, but in his or her social context, especially in his or her family environment. It is assumed that individual problems are often an expression of dysfunctional relationship patterns that have to be worked out and changed together.

An integrative approach draws on elements from different therapeutic schools to develop a tailor-made treatment concept that is tailored to the individual needs of the client.

The effectiveness of psychotherapy has been proven by numerous scientific studies. It not only promotes the management of symptoms such as anxiety, depression or compulsions, but also supports personal and social development. This is done by working on the relationship between therapist and client, exploring and understanding emotions, thoughts and behaviors, and promoting new coping strategies and approaches to life.

Psychotherapy is subject to ethical guidelines and requires sound training, continuous training and supervision of the therapist. A respectful, value-free and protected framework is essential so that the client can open up and work on his issues in a trusting manner. The aim is to provide the client with tools with which he can master his challenges independently.

Reactive attachment disorder of childhood

Reactive attachment disorder of childhood (RBS) is a severe but relatively rare disorder that is classified in the literature as an early childhood developmental disorder. It occurs in children who have experienced extreme neglect or abuse in early childhood. This severe emotional neglect or lack of a stable caregiver can affect a child's ability to develop secure and healthy attachments.

Characteristic of reactive attachment disorder are disorders in social relationship behavior, which can manifest themselves in different forms. Children with this disorder often show lower levels of social interaction. They have difficulty building and maintaining trusting relationships and often show ambivalent behavior towards caregivers.

A main characteristic of reactive attachment disorder is a clearly disturbed attachment behavior. Affected children often seem emotionally withdrawn and avoid closeness or seek it in an unusual way. They can fluctuate between a contradictory and insecure attachment and an overall disorganized lack of attachment. While some children avoid social interactions altogether or behave indifferently, others seek closeness irregularly but at the same time show signs of distrust or fear of caregivers.

Children with reactive attachment disorder also often exhibit behavioral problems such as aggressive behavior, outbursts of anger, as well as a lack of social reciprocity, which means that they have difficulty understanding social interactions and responding appropriately to them. In extreme cases, the lack of a secure attachment can lead to severe psycho-emotional problems, which manifest themselves in inner restlessness, reactive depression or psychosomatic complaints.

The diagnosis of reactive attachment disorder requires a precise clinical evaluation, which includes a comprehensive analysis of the child's development and previous relationship experiences. The diagnostic criterion here is not only on the current pattern of behavior, but also on the history of neglect and abuse in early childhood.

Treatment options for reactive attachment disorder usually include some form of trauma therapy, couples therapy or family therapy approaches that aim to catch up on secure attachment experiences. This can include working with foster parents, adoptive parents, or other stable caregivers. In addition, interventions are necessary that aim to gradually build and stabilize the child's trust and emotional bond.

When children with childhood reactive attachment disorder experience early therapeutic intervention and stable, reliable attachments, they can often show significant improvements in their social and emotional well-being. Nevertheless, reactive attachment disorder remains a serious and profound disorder that requires a high level of empathetic and specific therapeutic care.

Receptive speech disorder

A receptive language disorder, also known as speech comprehension disorder or speech comprehension disorder, is an impairment of the understanding of spoken or written language. People affected by this disorder have difficulty grasping the meanings of words, sentences, or more complex linguistic constructs. This can occur regardless of the ability to speak, which is why sufferers often speak normally or even above average, but without actually understanding what they are being told.

Children with receptive language disorders usually have problems interpreting linguistic inputs correctly. This is often reflected in misunderstandings of requests and explanations. They may have difficulty following instructions, retelling stories, or answering questions correctly. For example, if a teacher gives an instruction, the child may not understand that instruction correctly and therefore will not be able to perform the expected action. In a social context, this can easily lead to misunderstanding and isolation, as it makes it difficult to interact with peers and adults.

The causes of a receptive speech disorder are manifold. They can be genetic or occur as a result of developmental disorders such as autism or Down syndrome. Brain injuries, for example due to traumatic brain injury or infections of the central nervous system, can also lead to this disorder. Early childhood support deficits, especially in the linguistic and social areas, are also considered risk factors.

A receptive language disorder is usually diagnosed by professionals such as speech therapists, psychologists and pediatricians. To this end, standardised tests and informal assessment methods are used to determine language comprehension compared to the age norm. Often, the expressive language ability, i.e. the ability to pronounce and produce words, is also examined in the diagnosis in order to obtain a more comprehensive picture of the language skills of the person concerned.

Therapeutically, a multimodal approach is in the foreground. Speech therapy aims to expand vocabulary and promote the understanding of linguistic structures. Visual aids and games are often used to support the learning process. In some cases, it is also advisable to work with occupational therapists and psychologists to address concomitant disorders such as attention deficits or social anxiety. Parents and educators are often involved in therapy to ensure continuous support outside of therapy sessions.

In the long term, the goal is to help those affected to participate as well as possible in everyday life and social interactions. The prognosis varies depending on the severity of the disorder and the individual conditions. Early diagnosis and intervention usually increase the chances of significant improvements in language understanding.

Reframing

Reframing is a therapeutic procedure that is mainly used in cognitive behavioral therapy, systemic therapy and NLP (Neuro-Linguistic Programming). It describes the process of looking at a problem, situation, or experience from a new, different perspective, thereby changing the meaning that the problem has for the affected person. The aim of this approach is to modify the perception and emotional experience of the individual in order to enable beneficial behavioural changes and new possibilities for action.

In a therapeutic context, reframing is used to identify dysfunctional thought patterns and negative interpretations of events and replace them with alternative, more positive and helpful perspectives. The therapist supports the client in loosening rigid beliefs and entrenched views by using various techniques and questions. These include:

- Targeted questions: Through targeted questions, the therapist can help the client to question his or her own perception and gain new insights. Examples include: "What positive aspects could be hidden in this situation?" or "How would someone you admire see this situation?"
- Change of perspective: The therapist encourages the client to look at the situation from different angles, e.g. from the point of view of an uninvolved observer or by a time shift by asking how the client would evaluate the event in retrospect in a year.
- Change of meaning: Through communication and targeted interventions, the therapist can help find new meanings for stressful events or experiences. A negative experience, for example, can be reinterpreted as an important learning experience.

Reframing can be effective on both a mental and emotional level. By changing the cognitive representation of a stressful situation, the emotional response of the affected person can also change. In the long term, this often leads to increased problem-solving skills and self-efficiency, as the client learns to react more flexibly to challenges and to consider different interpretations.

A practical example of reframing could be a client who sees a termination as a personal defeat and disaster. Through therapeutic reframing, resignation could be interpreted as an opportunity to explore new professional opportunities, pursue personal interests, or use valuable time off for reflection and reorientation. This new perspective can reduce the negative emotions associated with quitting while promoting positive motivation and confidence.

Relapse prevention

In psychotherapy, relapse prevention refers to a variety of measures aimed at preventing the recurrence of mental illnesses or symptoms after successful treatment. This term is particularly relevant in the treatment of chronic or recurrent mental disorders such as depression, anxiety disorders, schizophrenia or addictions.

A central component of relapse prevention is psychoeducation. Those affected and often their relatives are informed about the nature of their illness, typical triggers and early warning signs of a relapse, and effective coping strategies. This knowledge enables patients to recognize signs of relapse early on and to act accordingly.

Another important aspect of relapse prevention is the development of individual coping strategies. Patients learn to identify stressful situations and potential triggers for their symptoms and to take targeted measures to reduce stress or avoid these triggers. Such measures may include mindfulness techniques, relaxation techniques, physical activity, or healthy eating.

The regularity of therapeutic sessions, even after the intensive treatment has been completed, can be a significant factor. These sessions provide a space for reflection, clarification of emerging issues and reinforcement of coping mechanisms that have already been learned.

Medical support plays a decisive role in many cases. Patients taking medication to stabilize their mental health benefit from continuous collaboration with their treating physician to determine the optimal dosage and possible adjustments. Regular medical follow-up appointments can help to monitor side effects and adapt long-term treatment to the individual clinical picture.

Social support, whether through family, friends or self-help groups, is an additional key factor in relapse prevention. A strong social network can provide emotional support and help prevent isolation, which is often a risk of relapse.

After all, self-management plays an essential role in relapse prevention. It promotes personal responsibility and self-efficacy in those affected. By keeping a symptom diary, where mood, thoughts and behaviors are noted, patterns and early warning signs can be made visible. At the first signs of a possible relapse, influence and action can then be taken before it deteriorates.

Resilience

Resilience refers to an individual's ability to successfully deal with and cope with stress, adversity and traumatic events. It is a dynamic concept that includes psychological, social and biological factors. Resilience does not mean merely persevering or passively persevering, but rather the active and positive cultivation of coping strategies that enable the person to remain healthy and functional despite stress.

On a psychological level, the inner attitude plays a central role. People who are considered resilient often have a high degree of self-efficacy and optimism. They are able to accept challenges as part of life and learn from them. This attitude allows them to get back up and move on faster after setbacks.

Another central aspect of resilience is the ability to self-regulate. Resilient people can consciously control and adapt their emotions, thoughts and behaviors in order to adapt flexibly to different situations. They have good problem-solving skills and are able to find alternative ways when a plan fails.

Social support also plays an essential role in developing and maintaining resilience. Close relationships with family, friends, or community members provide emotional support and foster a sense of belonging and security. These social networks act as a buffer against stress and help to better process stressful experiences.

Biological factors, such as genetic makeup and neurobiological mechanisms, can also influence resilience. For example, it has been shown that certain genes and the interaction of neurotransmitters can influence stress responses and emotional regulation. However, this does not mean that resilience is exclusively biologically determined; the interaction with environmental factors is crucial.

Furthermore, life history plays an important role in the development of resilience. Previous experience with coping behavior and success in overcoming difficulties contribute to the development of a repertoire of adaptive strategies. Traumatic experiences in childhood can also lead to increased vulnerabilities on the one hand, but on the other hand they can also form the basis for the development of strong resilience if they are mitigated by supportive relationship experiences.

In psychotherapy, the promotion of resilience can be a central therapeutic goal. Therapists work to strengthen their clients' self-efficacy, develop adaptive coping strategies, and mobilize the social network. Various therapeutic approaches such as cognitive behavioral therapy, mindfulness and acceptance-based procedures and systemic therapy offer different tools to specifically promote resilience.

Resistance

Resistance is a central concept in psychotherapy, originally introduced by Sigmund Freud in psychoanalysis and still plays a significant role in various therapeutic approaches today. It refers to the unconscious defense mechanisms and conscious actions or attitudes of a patient that are directed against the progress of the therapy and hinder or delay the therapeutic process.

This term encompasses a wide range of phenomena. Sometimes resistance manifests itself very subtly, for example by forgetting therapy appointments, digressing in conversations or avoiding certain topics. In other cases, it can also occur more obviously, for example through direct rejection of therapeutic interventions or even discontinuation of therapy.

The causes of resistance are manifold. They are often based on a fear of change, as therapeutic processes can bring painful emotions or repressed memories to light. The patient could unconsciously feel that uncovering certain topics opens up old wounds or questions the previous way of life. Resistance can also be an expression of a lack of trust in the therapist or in the therapeutic method. Furthermore, deeply rooted habits and beliefs often play a role, making it difficult to integrate new ways of thinking and behaving.

For the therapist, it is essential to understand resistance not only as an obstacle, but also as valuable information and an inevitable part of the therapeutic process. Resistance often reveals central conflicts and fears of the patient and, if understood and addressed, can pave the way to profound insights and change. The therapist must show a high degree of sensitivity and patience in order to carefully explore and work on the resistance without overtaxing the patient or jeopardizing the therapeutic relationship.

In concrete practice, the therapist has various techniques at his disposal to deal with resistance. This includes, among other things, careful confrontation, i.e. lovingly pointing out and questioning the patient's contradictory behaviors. Paradoxical interventions, in which the therapist recommends that the patient actively increase resistance, can also be effective. It is always important to have an appreciative and non-judgmental attitude that allows the patient to feel safe and understood.

Rett syndrome

Rett syndrome is a neurodevelopmental disorder that occurs almost exclusively in girls and is caused by mutations in the MECP2 gene on the X chromosome. These genetic changes lead to a malfunction of the protein MeCP2, which plays a central role in the regulation of gene expression. This results in a disorder of brain development and associated neurological abilities.

The course of Rett syndrome is typically divided into four stages. In the first phase, which occurs between the ages of about 6 and 18 months, the affected children initially appear to develop normally. This phase is often referred to as the "quiet period". This is followed by a phase of rapid developmental standstill, in which the children lose existing skills such as speaking and the purposeful use of their hands. This regression is usually accompanied by characteristic hand stereotypes, such as hand wringing or hand washing, as well as reduced motor control.

The third phase, known as the plateau phase, usually occurs at preschool age. During this phase, some of the motor and communication skills stabilize, but the neurological impairments remain. Seizures, breathing disorders and scoliotic changes in the spine often occur.

In the fourth phase, which concerns adolescence and adulthood, further motor deterioration becomes visible. Muscle stiffness and spasticity increase, and many sufferers suffer from problems such as severe scoliosis and generally reduced mobility. Cognitive functions usually remain severely impaired, although some individual skills such as eye movements can be used for communication.

Diagnostically, Rett syndrome is often identified by observation of clinical symptoms and genetic testing. There are no curative therapies for Rett syndrome, but a multidisciplinary approach to treatment can significantly improve quality of life. Therapies include physical therapy, occupational therapy, speech therapy, and drug treatment to control seizure disorders and muscle stiffness.

Psychotherapeutic care also plays an essential role, especially for the families of those affected. Stress and anxiety management strategies, resource strengthening and emotional support help to meet daily challenges and create a positive living environment.

Rett syndrome presents comprehensively challenging situations for those affected and their families by having a profound impact on various areas of life. In addition to medical and therapeutic care, the promotion of social participation and the creation of a support network are of great importance.

Revealing psychotherapy

Revealing psychotherapy is a therapeutic method that aims to bring to light a patient's unconscious conflicts, repressed memories, and hidden psychological processes. This form of therapy is based on the assumption that past events and inner conflicts hidden in the unconscious strongly influence the current behavior and experience of the individual and can often lead to mental disorders.

In contrast to symptom-oriented or supportive therapy methods, which are aimed at alleviating current symptoms, uncovering psychotherapy focuses on exploring the underlying causes of these symptoms. By identifying and making aware of these unconscious factors, patients can develop a deeper understanding of their own inner workings and experience healing.

A central element of uncovering psychotherapy is the detailed analysis and processing of previous experiences and relationships, especially those from childhood and early adolescence. These can be traumatic experiences, unresolved conflicts with parents or other important caregivers as well as repressed feelings and needs. Through various techniques such as free association, dream analysis and the processing of transference and countertransference processes, the therapist helps the patient to recognize and integrate these hidden contents.

An important technique in revealing psychotherapy is free association, in which the patient is encouraged to express his thoughts and feelings without censorship. This method allows spontaneous and often unexpected content from the unconscious to be brought to the surface. Working with dreams also plays an important role, as dreams are seen as an expression of unconscious desires, fears and conflicts.

The therapeutic relationship itself is also seen as an essential tool to make these deep inner processes accessible. The therapist provides a safe space where the patient can open up and confidently explore their innermost thoughts and feelings. Transference, the phenomenon in which the patient transfers feelings and ideas that were originally directed at important people in the past to the therapist, is actively used in revealing psychotherapy to recognize and work on these old patterns.

The path to healing in uncovering psychotherapy is often lengthy and challenging, as uncovering and working through deeper conflicts and traumatic experiences can cause painful feelings. However, it is precisely the confrontation with these aspects and the gradual integration into conscious experience that enables the patient to gain a deeper understanding of himself, which ultimately makes profound changes and healing possible.

Roleplaying game

Role-playing is a therapeutic method that is often used in psychotherapy to help clients better understand and work on their emotions and behaviors in specific situations. This approach comes from psychodrama therapy, which was developed by the Austrian psychiatrist Jacob Levy Moreno.

In role-playing, the clients slip into different roles, which can either represent their own or other characters. This allows them to put themselves in different perspectives and look at experiences and emotions from a new point of view.

A central component of role-playing is the re-enactment of situations that play an important role in the lives of the clients. This can be, for example, a conflict in the work environment, a family quarrel or a social interaction where the person feels difficulties. By actively acting out these scenarios, clients can test alternative behaviors and reactions without addressing the immediate consequences of these actions in real life.

Therapists guide role-play and ensure that clients feel safe and supported. The therapists' tasks include structuring the scenarios, asking questions and giving feedback so that clients can reflect on their experiences and learn from them.

Through role-playing, clients gain deeper insights into their own emotional triggers and reactions. You will have the opportunity to develop problem-solving strategies and learn new communication skills. In addition, role-playing can help to increase empathy towards other people by allowing them to understand their views and feelings.

Although role-play can be useful in many therapeutic contexts, it is especially valuable in treating social anxiety, relationship problems, and traumatic experiences. Here it serves as a safe space in which clients can work on difficult topics and challenges in a controlled environment.

Rorschach Test

The Rorschach test, also known as the Rorschach inkblot test, is a psychological projection method used in diagnostics and research. It was developed in 1921 by the Swiss psychiatrist Hermann Rorschach and is based on the analysis of responses to a series of symmetrical inkblot images.

The test consists of ten plates, each of which shows different types of ink blotches. These blobs can take on ambiguous, often complex forms that each viewer can interpret differently. When the test is carried out, the subject is shown each of the panels individually and is asked to say what he sees on them or what comes to mind. The answers are recorded or noted verbatim and then evaluated and analyzed according to certain criteria.

The interpretation of the results is based on various factors:

- **Content of the answers**: What does the test subject see in the ink blotches? These can be animals, people, objects or completely abstract shapes.

- **Location**: Which part of the blob is used to give the answer? This includes totalities, individual parts or details of the blob.

- **Determinants**: What aspects of the blob (shape, movement, color, shadow) influenced perception? This indicates the subject's cognitive and emotional processing.

- **Level of organization**: How well can the subject make a coherent and organized observation of the blob? This is seen as an indicator of the ability to structure reality.

The Rorschach test is often referred to as a projective procedure because it assumes that people project unconscious processes, desires, fears and deep-seated emotional conflicts when interpreting the ambiguous blobs. It is thus a means of gaining access to deep psychological structures that are difficult to grasp in standardized or directly interrogative tests.

Although the test is considered difficult to standardize due to its projective character and partly subjective in its interpretation, several standardized evaluation methods have developed that attempt to systematically and objectively code the answers.

Critics complain about the validity and reliability of the test, which means that the results cannot always be reliably repeated and the validity of the statements made about the personality of the test person is doubted. Nevertheless, the Rorschach Test continues to be used in clinical practice and psychological research, mainly due to its ability to shed light on deeply hidden and hard-to-reach areas of the psyche.

Rumble

Rumbling refers to a communication disorder in which the speed of speech is unusually high and the intelligibility of speech is significantly impaired. People who rumble often speak very quickly, which leads them to omit or merge sounds, syllables or whole words. As a result, the language often seems rushed and disorganized. Those affected often have difficulty maintaining the clarity of their statements and the structural integrity of their statements.

This disorder can occur in both children and adults and is usually diagnosed with the so-called stutter-rumble distinction. In contrast to stuttering, which is characterized by the frequent repetition of sounds or words as well as blockages and pauses, rumbling manifests itself primarily in fast and often chaotic speech. The person who rumbles is often unaware of the way they speak and has difficulty regulating the pace independently.

The causes of rumbling are diverse and not fully understood. It is assumed that neurophysiological, genetic and language development-related factors may play a role. In addition, psychological aspects, such as stress or an existing language development disorder, can also influence or intensify rumbling.

Rumbling is diagnosed by a comprehensive speech therapy and psychological analysis. Here, speech behavior is analyzed and documented. In addition to observing the speed of speech and speech intelligibility, anamnesis interviews and standardized test procedures are also important.

The therapy of rumbling usually aims to regulate the speed of speech and improve articulation. Various methods and techniques are used, such as speaking exercises to slow down the pace of speech, breathing and relaxation techniques as well as exercises to build up a more conscious feeling for language. The involvement of parents and teachers, especially with children, is also an important part of therapy to create a supportive environment.

In addition, working on self-perception plays a major role. Since many blusterers are not aware of their way of speaking, therapy often includes exercises to perceive and reflect on one's own speaking behavior. The aim is to help those affected to speak more consciously and controlled, which facilitates communication in everyday life and reduces misunderstandings.

Rumbling can also be treated with the help of group or individual therapies. In group therapies, those affected are given the opportunity to practice their communication skills in a social context and to collect feedback from others. Individual therapies, on the other hand, offer a more intensive and individual approach that is specifically tailored to the needs and challenges of the individual.

In addition, therapy can be supported by technological aids such as speech speed measuring devices or computer-aided speech programs. These help those affected to receive clearer feedback about their speech speed and quality and to consciously work on improvement.

The ultimate goal of treatment is to promote clear and understandable language that benefits both the person and those around them. Despite the challenges that rumbling can bring, many affected individuals show significant progress thanks to appropriate therapeutic measures and continuous support.

Schema therapy

Schema therapy is an integrative psychotherapy method developed by Jeffrey Young in the 1980s. It combines concepts and techniques from cognitive behavioral therapy, Gestalt therapy, attachment theory, psychoanalysis and emotion-focused therapy. The goal of schema therapy is to recognize and change deep-rooted patterns (schemata) and survival strategies that often developed in childhood and trigger problematic behaviors and emotions in adulthood.

Schemas are comprehensive cognitive and emotional patterns that result from early life experiences. They influence how people perceive themselves and others and how they react to their environment. These schemata can lead to recurring, destructive life patterns if not recognized and worked on. For example, the most common schemes include the abandonment scheme, the distrust scheme and the inadequacy scheme.

A central element of schema therapy is the concept of mode work. Here, a person's behavior is understood as an interplay of different emotional states or "modes". These modes represent different aspects of personality, such as "hurt child mode", "angry child mode", "critical parent mode" or healthy modes. By working with these emotional states, the understanding of the triggers and mechanisms of problematic behaviors is expanded and changes are sought.

In schema therapy, the therapeutic relationship plays a central role. It serves not only for conflict management, but also as a corrective experience. The therapist takes an active empathetic stance and provides support and affirmation to help the patient develop new, adaptive patterns of thought and behavior. The concept of limited post-parenting is also used here, in which the therapist becomes a kind of surrogate parent for the patient to satisfy emotional needs that remained unsatisfied in childhood.

Therapy often includes several phases: First, the existing schemes and modes are recorded and understood. In the subsequent change phase, new, healthier patterns of behavior and thinking are practiced. Finally, the consolidation phase follows, in which the new patterns are integrated into everyday life and sustainable changes in the patient's relationships and lifestyle habits are consolidated.

Schema therapy has proven to be particularly effective in the treatment of personality disorders, chronic depression, anxiety disorders and post-traumatic stress disorder. Through its integrative and depth-psychologically grounded approach, it offers a comprehensive opportunity to change deep-seated emotional problems and behavioral patterns in the long term.

Schizoid personality disorder

Schizoid personality disorder (SPS) is a mental illness characterized by a profound pattern of withdrawal from social relationships and limited expression of emotions in interpersonal contexts. People with this personality disorder often show little interest in close relationships, including family ties, and have difficulty enjoying social activities and interactions.

Affected persons often seem distant, introverted and emotionally cold, which is often interpreted as indifference to praise or criticism. They find it difficult to feel joy or enthusiasm for activities that many people experience as enjoyable or satisfying. This lack of affective reactivity can be particularly noticeable in interpersonal relationships, where they are often perceived as aloof or reserved.

Professionally and socially, individuals with PLCs tend to prefer activities that require little to no social interaction, as they are more comfortable in such environments. They are often able to think objectively and analytically, which can make them successful in certain professional fields where social skills are less prominent. Despite these functional adjustments, many sufferers subjectively feel like outsiders and have a limited number of close friendships or social ties.

A central characteristic of the schizoid personality is the low level of desire and joy in social interactions as well as in sensual pleasures. This can lead to those affected often being seen as loners who seek neither the closeness nor the warmth of other people. Sexual experiences are also often of little interest, which is not to be equated with a complete absence of sexuality, but can be interpreted as part of the general lack of pleasure.

With regard to the etiological aspects of SPS, it is assumed that both genetic and environmental factors play a role. Early attachment experiences and the emotional climate in the parental home can have a significant influence on the development of the disorder. Hypotheses include possible emotional neglect or lack of adequate emotional warmth in childhood.

People with PLD rarely seek therapeutic help on their own, often because they do not find their symptoms bothersome. However, when they enter therapy, an important treatment approach can be to help them overcome social isolation and strengthen emotional skills. Psychotherapeutic interventions can aim to promote awareness of emotions and learn techniques to improve relationships. However, a particular challenge remains to consolidate trust and motivation to participate in therapy.

Treatment can be complex and often requires a tailored, patient approach that respects the individual's idiosyncrasies and needs. Complementary treatments, such as socio-educational support or creative therapies, can also be useful in increasing social functioning levels and improving quality of life.

Schizophrenia

Schizophrenia is a severe mental disorder characterized by profound impairments in thinking, perception and emotional responsiveness. Typically, it manifests in late adolescence or early adulthood and can affect both men and women, with men often showing symptoms earlier than women.

A key feature of schizophrenia is psychosis, in which a person loses touch with reality. This often includes hallucinations, in which someone sees, hears, or feels things that only exist in their head, and delusions, which are entrenched false beliefs, even if they contradict reality or logical premises.

The symptoms of schizophrenia can be divided into three main categories:

1. **Positive symptoms**: These are excesses or distortions of normal functions. They include hallucinations, delusions, disorganized thinking and speech, and grossly disorganized or catatonic behavior.
2. **Negative symptoms**: These represent a deficit or loss of normal functions, such as affective flattening (lack of emotional expression), alogy (decreased speech production), asociality, anhedonia (inability to feel pleasure), and apathy.
3. **Cognitive symptoms**: Schizophrenia often affects memory, attention, and the ability to process information. Difficulties in performing everyday tasks, problems with understanding or decision-making, and reduced ability to concentrate are typical cognitive impairments.

The etiology of schizophrenia is multifactorial. Genetic predispositions play an important role; the risk of developing schizophrenia is significantly increased in individuals with first-degree relatives who are affected. Neurobiological factors are also thought to be involved, such as dopamine dysregulation and structural brain abnormalities. In addition, psychosocial factors, stressors and environmental factors can influence the development of the disease.

Diagnostic criteria for schizophrenia, as defined in the DSM-5 (Diagnostic and Statistical Manual of Mental Disorders) and ICD-10 (International Classification of Diseases), require the presence of certain symptoms over a period of at least six months, with at least one month of active symptoms.

The treatment of schizophrenia requires a holistic approach that includes both drug and psychosocial interventions. Antipsychotic medications are fundamental to reducing positive symptoms. Psychosocial interventions such as cognitive behavioural therapy (CBT), social therapy measures and family interventions are also essential as they can improve the social functioning and quality of life of affected persons. Rehabilitation and integration programmes help those affected to lead as independent a life as possible again and to integrate into society.

The management of the disease requires a long-term commitment and close cooperation between psychotherapists, psychiatrists, social workers, relatives and the affected persons themselves.

Self-instruction training

Self-instruction training is a psychotherapeutic method that aims to modify a person's internal language and self-directed instructions in order to improve their behavior and cognitive processes. This technique is based on the assumption that the way people talk to themselves – their inner dialogues and self-talk – has a significant influence on their feelings and behavior.

Self-instruction training plays a central role in cognitive behavioral therapy and other cognitive-behavioral approaches. It assumes that dysfunctional self-instructions, such as negative self-evaluations or destructive thought patterns, contribute to emotional and behavioral problems. Through targeted training, these negative self-talk is replaced by constructive and helpful instructions.

A typical process in self-instruction training involves several steps:

1. Identification of dysfunctional self-instructions:

The first step is to recognize the negative or obstructive inner statements that a person gives to themselves. These can be conscious or unconscious and include self-criticism, pessimistic expectations or excessively strict self-evaluations.

2. Creation of new, functional self-instructions:

After identifying the negative self-instructions, new, positive and helpful self-instructions are formulated. These new instructions are intended to be realistic, motivating and supportive and can be developed step by step and checked in therapy.

3. **Training and application of the new self-instructions:**

The person is guided to consciously use the new self-instructions in different situations. This can be done through role-playing, behavioral exercises, and repeated practice. It makes sense to initially choose simple and less stressful situations and gradually move towards more complex or emotionally challenging scenarios.

4. **Evaluation and adaptation:**

The effectiveness of the new self-instructions is regularly reviewed. Feedback loops allow instructions to be modified and further adjusted as needed to ensure they are effective and helpful.

Through self-instruction training, patients can learn to consciously control their inner language and thus regulate their thoughts and emotions. This can lead to an improvement in self-control and self-efficacy and help to reduce dysfunctional behavior patterns.

This training has proven to be especially useful in treating anxiety disorders, depression, ADHD, and other mental health issues. When dealing with stressful or challenging situations, the techniques learned can help to strengthen a person's resilience and promote their psychological well-being.

Sense of coherence

The sense of coherence is a central concept within salutogenesis, a concept developed by Aaron Antonovsky that deals with the conditions and processes of the emergence of health. The sense of coherence describes a person's individual ability to experience their life as understandable, manageable and meaningful, even in times of stress and strain. It is made up of three main components: comprehensibility, manageability and meaningfulness.

Comprehensibility refers to the extent to which a person perceives the events and developments in their life as ordered, structured, and predictable. People with a high degree of comprehension tend to experience the world as coherent and not chaotic. They feel able to cognitively grasp and explain events. This gives them a sense of control and predictability, even if not all the details are known.

Manageability is the conviction that you have enough resources at your disposal to meet the demands of life. These resources can be internal in nature, such as skills and abilities, or external, such as social support and financial resources. People who feel a high degree of manageability believe that they can cope with life's challenges. They feel empowered to respond actively and successfully to stressors and problems.

Meaningfulness encompasses the extent to which a person perceives life as emotionally and existentially meaningful. This component emphasizes the importance of commitment and associated feelings of joie de vivre and contentment. People with a high degree of meaningfulness feel anchored in their existence and see a deeper meaning in their activities and relationships, which helps them to accept adversity as important and necessary parts of the path of life.

A strong sense of coherence is a major contributor to mental health, as it allows people to see challenges as manageable and meaningful. This reduces the subjective feeling of strain, and the level of stress can be lowered. A well-developed sense of coherence thus supports resilience and contributes to long-term psychological stability and well-being.

Building and strengthening this sense of coherence can be an important goal within psychotherapy. Through the use of various therapeutic techniques and approaches, such as cognitive behavioral therapy or systemic therapy, clients can be supported to improve their understanding of the world, mobilize their resources and promote their purpose in life. A strong sense of coherence enables the individual not only to survive crises, but also to learn from them and emerge internally strengthened.

Sensory illusions or perceptual illusions

Sensory illusions, also known as perceptual illusions, refer to phenomena in which the sensory information of the individual is misinterpreted so that the perception does not correspond to the objective reality. Such delusions can affect all the senses – sight, hearing, smell, taste and touch – and manifest in various forms, often as hallucinations or illusions.

A hallucination is a special type of perceptual illusion in which a person experiences the strongest sensory impressions even though there is no real external source of stimuli. These can be visual (seeing non-existent people or objects), auditory (hearing voices or sounds that do not exist), olfactory (smelling non-existent scents or stench), gustatory (tasting non-existent substances), or tactile (feeling non-existent touch or insects on the skin). Hallucinations can occur in severe psychiatric disorders, such as schizophrenia, as well as in physical illnesses, such as epilepsy or brain disorders. They can also be caused by drug use or withdrawal.

Illusions, on the other hand, are misperceptions in which an existing stimulus is interpreted in a distorted way. A classic example would be the phenomenon of mistakeing a tree stump for a wild animal in a shady piece of forest. Here, the sensory input is real, but the interpretation of what is perceived is flawed. Illusions are common and usually harmless unless they lead to dangerous misconduct.

The causes of sensory illusions can be manifold. They can be caused by neuronal dysfunction, mental illness, the influence of psychoactive substances or sensory deprivation. Certain neurological conditions such as migraines, epilepsy or strokes can also alter sensory perception, often associated with specific sensory aura phenomena.

From the perspective of psychotherapy, understanding and distinguishing sensory illusions is essential for diagnosis and the choice of therapeutic approaches. It is essential to take a thorough medical history to understand the nature and origin of sensory illusion and to distinguish between pathological and non-pathological forms. For example, a patient who reports auditory hallucinations may need a different therapeutic approach than someone who experiences optical illusions in anxiety-inducing situations.

Both drug and psychotherapeutic interventions play a role in treatment. While antipsychotics can work for hallucinatory states, cognitive behavioral therapy and other psychotherapeutic methods can help improve the interpretation and management of illusions.

The diagnostic criteria and treatment recommendations for sensory illusions are described in detail in specialist literature and diagnostic manuals, such as the DSM-5 (Diagnostic and Statistical Manual of Mental Disorders) and the ICD-10 (International Classification of Diseases), and should always be compared with current scientific findings.

Sexual dysfunction

Sexual dysfunction refers to a group of problems that affect a person's ability to experience sexual arousal or satisfaction. These disorders can occur in both men and women and vary significantly in their nature and influence. They encompass a variety of symptoms and are often to be considered interdisciplinary, as they have both psychological and physical dimensions.

Sexual dysfunction can be divided into different categories. A widely used classification includes:

1. **Desire disorders**: This is a decreased interest in sexual activity. People with this disorder have little to no sexual imagination and show little desire for sexual interaction. Examples include hypoactive sexual desire and sexual aversion.
2. **Arousal disorders**: These include difficulty achieving or maintaining sexual arousal. In women, this can manifest as a lack of genital or subjective arousal. Men may have difficulty getting or maintaining an erection (erectile dysfunction).
3. **Orgasm disorders**: These affect the inability to reach orgasm despite sufficient sexual arousal. Women may have difficulty experiencing a climax, while men

may sometimes have a premature or delayed orgasm.
4. **Pain disorders**: These include disorders such as dyspareunia (painful sexual intercourse) and vaginismus (involuntary contractions of the vaginal muscles that make sexual intercourse painful or impossible).

The causes of sexual dysfunction are varied and can be psychological, physical or social in nature. Psychological factors include anxiety, depression, stress, low self-esteem, or traumatic experiences. Physical causes can include hormonal imbalances, neurological disorders, chronic diseases, or the side effects of certain medications. Social and cultural factors, including relationship problems, communication difficulties, and societal taboos, also play an important role.

Diagnostic procedures require a comprehensive medical history that takes into account both the medical and psychosocial history of the person concerned. Sensitivity and discretion are important here in order to create a trusting environment in which the patient can talk openly about his problems.

Therapeutic approaches vary depending on the cause and severity of sexual dysfunction. Cognitive behavioral therapy, couples therapy and sex therapy are frequently used psychotherapeutic methods. Drug treatments, hormonal therapies or mechanical aids can also be part of a comprehensive treatment plan.

Sleep disorder

Sleep disorders, also known as insomnia, are common and widespread complaints in the field of psychotherapy and general medicine. They affect the quality, quantity and timing of sleep and often cause considerable stress and restrictions in the everyday life of those affected. Sleep disorders can occur in different forms and intensities, ranging from occasional problems falling asleep to chronic insomnia.

A fundamental characteristic of sleep disorders is the inability to get enough restorative sleep. This can manifest itself in someone having difficulty falling asleep, waking up several times during the night and having difficulty falling back asleep, or waking up early in the morning without the ability to fall asleep again. The consequences of sleep disorders are often felt during the day and include increased fatigue, concentration and memory problems, irritable mood, reduced performance and increased emotional and physical stress.

Causes of sleep disorders are diverse and can include both physical and psychological factors. The most common physical causes include sleep apnea, restless legs syndrome, chronic pain, and certain neurological or endocrine disorders. Psychological causes are often stress, anxiety disorders, depression, bipolar disorder or trauma. In addition, lifestyle factors such as irregular sleep habits, excessive consumption of caffeine or alcohol, shift work or insufficient physical exercise may play a role.

In psychotherapeutic practice, the diagnosis of sleep disorders is an important step. This includes a detailed medical history that captures sleep patterns, lifestyle, emotional and physical health, and any medications and substances that may have been used. Therapists often use sleep logs or diaries and questionnaires to record sleep habits and disorders in detail.

Treatment for sleep disorders depends on the underlying causes and the specific nature of the disorder. Therapeutic approaches may include cognitive behavioral therapy for insomnia (CBT-I), relaxation techniques, sleep hygiene counseling, and medication if necessary. CBT-I is particularly effective and involves learning techniques for changing dysfunctional thoughts and behaviors related to sleep, promoting sleep hygiene, and developing consistent sleep patterns.

Sleep hygiene includes, among other things, maintaining a regular sleep schedule, creating a relaxing sleep environment, avoiding stimulants and activities before bed, and promoting a healthy lifestyle with a balanced diet and regular physical activity.

Sleep phases

Sleep phases refer to the different stages that a person goes through during sleep. These phases are part of a cycle that usually lasts 90 to 110 minutes and is repeated several times a night. A complete sleep cycle consists of several sleep phases that can be distinguished in their activity in the brain and body and fall into two main categories: non-REM sleep (NREM) and REM sleep (rapid eye movement).

Non-REM Sleep

1. **Phase N1 (falling asleep phase):** In this phase, the sleeper is in a transitional state between wakefulness and sleep. Muscle activity decreases, and muscle twitches occasionally occur. This phase is relatively short, accounting for about 5% of total sleep.
2. **Phase N2 (light sleep):** In this phase, the sleeping person is no longer consciously awake. The body temperature drops, and the heart rate slows down. This phase takes up a larger part of the sleep cycle, about 45-55%. Specific EEG patterns occur, including sleep spindles and K-complexes, which serve as responses to external sounds.
3. **Phase N3 (deep sleep or delta sleep):** This phase is characterized by the predominance of slow, high-amplitude delta waves in the EEG. During deep sleep, physical recovery takes place, the immune system is strengthened, and cell growth is promoted. This phase accounts for about 15-25% of nightly sleep and is considered particularly restorative and regenerative.

REM Sleep

This is the stage of sleep when dreaming is most intense and common. It accounts for about 20-25% of total sleep and becomes longer and more intense as the night progresses. REM sleep is characterized by rapid eye movements, increased brain activity similar to wakefulness, and temporary muscle paralysis (atonia). This muscular atonia prevents the sleeper from physically living out his dreams. REM sleep plays an important role in the processing of emotions, memory, and cognitive processing.

Sleep phases are essential for overall physical and mental health. Disturbances in any of these stages can lead to various health problems, including insomnia, sleep apnea, and other sleep disorders. A good mix and the right sequence of these sleep phases are crucial for restful sleep and general well-being.

Social history

The social anamnesis is an essential part of psychotherapeutic diagnostics and refers to the systematic recording of the social living conditions and the life history of the patient. The aim is to gain a comprehensive picture of the social and interpersonal influences on the patient's life. This allows the therapist to identify the individual psychosocial factors that could contribute to the emergence and maintenance of mental health problems.

The social anamnesis typically covers several central subject areas:

1. Family history:

Here, the family structure, family relationships and family conflicts are recorded. Questions can relate to upbringing, traumatic experiences, relationships with parents and siblings, as well as family illnesses or entanglements. The therapist gains insight into the child's developmental conditions and family behavior patterns that may have a pathogenic effect or represent protective factors.

2. Educational and professional history:

This section deals with the patient's educational and professional development. These include school and vocational training, professional successes and failures, job changes as well as current professional situation and satisfaction. Conflicts at work, bullying or unemployment are also addressed here, as they represent potential stressors that can influence the patient's mental state.

3. Partnership and relationship history:

This is about the current and past partnerships and their qualities. The therapist examines the extent to which stable or unstable relationships, separations, divorces or the loss of a partner influence the psychological state. The patient's sexuality and any sexual problems or traumas are also addressed.

4. Social network and support system:

This section deals with the patient's wider social environment, including friends, neighbors, colleagues, and other important caregivers. The extent to which these people are perceived as supportive or stressful is examined. The therapist determines which social resources and networks are available to the patient that can be included or strengthened in therapy.

5. Housing and living situation:

This category lists information about the current place of residence, housing conditions and their stability. Particularly relevant here are possible housing problems, loneliness or the frequency of changes of residence, which could be psychological stressors.

6. Leisure behaviour and hobbies:

The patient's leisure activities, including hobbies, sports activities, and cultural interests, are also part of the social history. The therapist looks at activities that contribute to recovery and stress reduction and examines the extent to which the patient has a good work-life balance.

7. Financial situation:

The patient's economic situation can also have a significant impact on mental well-being. Debts, precarious employment or unexpected financial burdens are discussed in this context.

The detailed survey of these different aspects of life allows the therapist to place the patient's psychological issues in a larger social context. This comprehensive view not only facilitates the understanding of the current complaints, but also the development of individual therapeutic approaches tailored to the patient's specific life situation.

Social phobia

Social phobia, also known as social anxiety disorder, is a mental illness characterized by an intense fear of social situations or performance demands in which the person is exposed to possible evaluation by others. Those affected fear being judged, criticized or exposed negatively and usually react with excessive fear, severe discomfort or pronounced avoidance of these situations.

People with social anxiety often feel anxiety in everyday social interactions, such as speaking in public, participating in class or team discussions, eating or drinking in front of others, or meeting new people. This fear is often related to the worry of attracting embarrassment, appearing clumsy or being perceived as incompetent. At the core of these fears is the expectation of being negatively judged by others.

The symptoms of social phobia can be both psychological and physical. Psychologically, those affected experience intense anxiety days or weeks before the event (anticipatory fear), they have negative or obsessive thoughts about the upcoming situation and tend to devalue their own social skills. Physical symptoms may include trembling, sweating, redness, palpitations, nausea, or difficulty breathing.

These anxiety symptoms often lead to serious avoidance behavior. Those affected consistently avoid situations that trigger anxiety or only endure them under great tension and with considerable inner resistance. However, continued avoidance intensifies the phobia because the affected person has no opportunity to learn that their fears are mostly unfounded.

The socio-economic and personal effects of social phobia are significant. Career opportunities, educational and relationship opportunities can be severely limited. This, in turn, can lead to further withdrawal, isolation, and, in severe cases, the development of comorbid disorders such as depression or substance abuse.

The causes of social phobia are multifactorial. Genetic predispositions, neurobiological factors, and personal experiences such as bullying, excessive criticism, or traumatic social events may play a role. Certain personality traits such as increased shyness or reluctance in childhood can also increase the risk.

The treatment of social phobia usually involves a combination of psychotherapeutic methods, pharmacotherapy and self-help strategies. Cognitive behavioral therapy (CBT) is particularly effective in this regard. It helps those affected to identify and change irrational thought patterns and to gradually confront fearful situations. In addition, medications such as selective serotonin reuptake inhibitors (SSRIs) can be used to relieve symptoms. Social skills training and exposure therapy are also therapeutic approaches that can help.

Social Skills Training

Social Competence Training (SKT) is a structured program within psychotherapy that aims to improve social skills and interpersonal communication skills. It is often aimed at people who have difficulty interacting with others, whether due to social anxiety, autism spectrum disorders, ADHD, or other mental and psychosocial issues. The training aims to increase the ability of those affected to behave safely and appropriately in social situations.

The first step in social competence training is to diagnose and identify specific deficits. The diagnostic phase can be carried out through structured interviews, questionnaires or behavioral observations. Important social skills that could be addressed in the training include initiating and maintaining conversations, expressing feelings, setting boundaries, and accepting feedback.

The training itself is practice-oriented and uses a variety of methods and techniques. Role-playing is one of the central methods; participants slip into different social roles and practice specific social scenarios. These role-playing games provide a safe environment in which mistakes can be made and corrected. Video feedback can also be used, where participants view and analyze their own social interactions, which also leads to a better understanding of their own social behaviors.

Another important aspect is the teaching of social-cognitive skills such as perspective-taking and empathy. Here we will discuss how to better understand and predict the thoughts and feelings of other people. Methods such as thought experiments and guided imagination can help to sharpen empathy.

Training in concrete social skills is often supported by model learning. Here, a goal-oriented behavior is demonstrated by the therapist and then practiced imitatively by the participants. This can include, for example, how to express constructive criticism or de-escalate conflicts. Non-verbal communication is often also worked on, such as eye contact, body language and tone of voice.

Another aspect of SKT is the application of the skills learned in everyday life. This is done through so-called transfer tasks, in which the participants are instructed to visit specific social situations outside of the training sessions and apply the skills they have learned there. The experiences will be reflected on in the next meeting and, if necessary, readjusted.

Social skills training can take place in both individual and group settings. A group setting has the advantage that the participants can learn from each other and a realistic social environment is offered. There are also programs that are tailored to specific age groups, such as children and adolescents, or to specific disorders.

Somatization disorder

Somatization disorder is a chronic mental illness characterized by the recurrence of a variety of physical complaints that cannot be fully supported by a medical explanation. People who suffer from this disorder often experience a variety of symptoms that can affect different body systems, including muscle pain, gastrointestinal discomfort, headaches, and sexual dysfunction.

Those affected often perceive their symptoms as very stressful and impairing. They often seek medical help and undergo numerous diagnostic tests and medical examinations, which, however, usually remain without clear organic findings. This leads to a high degree of frustration and despair among both those affected and the treating physicians.

The cause of somatization disorder is multifactorial. There is evidence that both genetic and psychosocial factors may play a role. Those affected often have a history of traumatic experiences or stressful life events and often have an increased sensitivity to physical sensations. This sensitivity can lead to increased perception and interpretation of normal physical signals as signs of serious illness.

Models of learning theory can also contribute to the explanation. For example, patients may have learned that physical complaints involve attention and care from other people, as well as relief from demands and obligations.

Diagnostically, the somatization disorder is listed among the somatic stress disorders in the DSM-5 (Diagnostic and Statistical Manual of Mental Disorders). It is characteristic that the symptoms are taken very seriously despite the lack of organic findings and are not dismissed as imaginary. Psychotherapists work to support those affected in dealing with the symptoms and to develop alternative coping strategies.

The treatment of somatization disorder requires a multidisciplinary approach. Effective therapy may include cognitive behavioral therapy (CBT), which aims to identify and change patients' maladaptive thought patterns and behaviors. In addition, psychoeducation can help those affected to develop a better understanding of the connections between body and psyche. In some cases, drug treatment, such as antidepressants, may also be indicated to relieve comorbid depression or anxiety.

Since the disorder is chronic, a long-term treatment approach is necessary.

Somatoform autonomic dysfunction

Somatoform autonomic dysfunction (SAFS) is a specific form of somatoform disorder in which patients experience physical symptoms that indicate dysfunction of the autonomic nervous system, without an organic cause being found. These symptoms typically affect the cardiovascular, gastrointestinal, respiratory or genitourinary systems and are often an expression of psychological stress.

Patients with SAFS experience a variety of symptoms that can be interpreted as an expression of malfunction of the autonomic nervous system. They often report tachycardia, chest pain, shortness of breath, dizziness, gastrointestinal problems such as nausea or diarrhea, and genitourinary symptoms such as a frequent urge to urinate. These complaints can vary greatly and often occur in connection with stressful situations or emotional difficulties.

A central feature of SAFS is the lack of organic findings. Despite extensive medical examinations, no physiological cause for the symptoms can be found. This often leads to frustration for both patients and treating physicians, as the symptoms are real and distressing, yet no tangible physical cause can be found.

The development of SAFS is multifactorial and often a combination of genetic dispositions, psychological factors and stress. Psychodynamic theories indicate that the physical symptoms can be seen as an expression of unconscious conflicts or as a form of communication of psychological suffering. Cognitive-behavioral approaches emphasize the role of erroneous perceptions and reinforcement mechanisms, in which everyday body sensations are interpreted as threatening and thus reinforced.

The treatment of SAFS requires a multimodal therapy concept. Psychotherapeutic interventions, especially cognitive behavioral therapy (CBT), have proven effective. These forms of therapy help patients to recognize the connection between psychological stress and physical symptoms and to develop adequate coping strategies. In addition, relaxation techniques such as progressive muscle relaxation or mindfulness exercises can help to alleviate physical symptoms and calm the autonomic nervous system.

Pharmacotherapy can be used as a supplement, especially if a comorbid depressive or anxiety disorder is present. Antidepressants or anxiolytic medications can help stabilize the general mental state and reduce the intensity of the symptoms.

Somatoform disorder

Somatoform disorder refers to a class of mental disorders in which affected individuals experience physical symptoms that may have a medical basis but cannot be fully explained by a medical illness or substance exposure. These symptoms cause significant suffering or significantly impair the everyday life of those affected.

The most common physical symptoms include pain, gastrointestinal complaints, sexual problems and pseudoneurological symptoms (e.g. fainting spells or paralysis). These symptoms often vary in location and intensity and can persist over a longer period of time or occur episodic.

A somatoform disorder can be divided into several subcategories, including:

1. **Somatization disorder**: Characterized by a variety of physical complaints that have existed for years and affect various organ systems and cannot be fully explained by a medical disease.
2. **Undifferentiated somatization disorder**: In this case, fewer and less complex symptoms occur than in the classic somatization disorder, but they last at least six months.
3. **Hypochondriacal disorder**: Sufferers suffer from the persistent belief or strong fear that they are suffering from a serious illness or that they are already ill, even

though medical examinations do not provide sufficient findings.
4. **Pain disorder**: The primary symptom is persistent pain in one or more parts of the body that cannot be explained solely by a medical condition. Psychological factors play an important role in the development and maintenance of pain.
5. **Conversion disorder (dissociative disorders):** Neurological symptoms such as paralysis, movement disorders or sensory changes are experienced that cannot be explained by neurological or other medical findings.

The development of somatoform disorders can be attributed to various causes, including genetic predispositions, neurobiological factors, early childhood attachment experiences, traumatic experiences, unfavorable family circumstances and chronic stress. A maladaptive approach to physical sensations and unfavorable disease models also play a central role.

Various methods are available in therapy. Cognitive behavioral therapy (CBT) has been shown to be effective in helping patients change dysfunctional thoughts and behavior patterns. In addition, techniques for stress management and relaxation are taught.

In addition to CBT, body-oriented procedures such as physiotherapy and biofeedback can also have a supportive effect. Multidisciplinary approaches, where physicians, psychologists, and physiotherapists work together, can be particularly efficient. Promoting the doctor-patient relationship is also crucial to building trust and increasing compliance. The goal is to help patients better understand

and manage their symptoms without constantly seeking medical explanations or investigations.

Somnambulism

Somnambulism, commonly known as sleepwalking, refers to a sleep disorder that belongs to the group of parasomnias. This disorder typically occurs during the so-called non-REM sleep phase, especially in the deeper stages of sleep, when the person sleeps hard and is difficult to wake up. This condition is characterized by the fact that the affected person gets out of bed asleep and performs simple to complex activities without having full consciousness or memory.

During an episode of somnambulism, the sufferer may exhibit simple actions such as getting up and walking around, or more complex behavioral patterns such as opening doors, putting on clothes, or even driving. The movements are often rather mechanical and automated, and the affected person shows reduced responsiveness and limited fine motor skills. Although the eyes are often open and have a glassy, staring expression, the person is usually unable to respond adequately to external stimuli or remember the events of the episode.

Somnambulism is more common in children than adults, and in some cases can be accompanied by other sleep disorders, such as night terrors (pavor nocturnus) or restless sleep patterns. The exact mechanism behind somnambulism is not yet fully understood, but various factors, including genetic predispositions, sleep deprivation, fever, stress, and certain medications, can favor the occurrence of such episodes.

The diagnosis of somnambulism is usually made through a thorough medical history and, if necessary, polysomnography, which analyzes the sleep architecture of the affected person. This examination helps to rule out other disorders and identify the specific pattern of sleep activity that leads to the somnambulistic episodes.

Treatment for somnambulism depends on the severity and frequency of episodes. For many children, somnambulism is a temporary phase that often passes without special treatment. Measures to improve sleep hygiene and relaxation techniques can be helpful in reducing the risk of episodes. In adults or severe cases, medication can also be considered that stabilizes sleep or modifies the deep sleep phases.

Special care should be taken when designing the sleeping environment to prevent injury during sleepwalking. This can include securing doors and windows, removing obstacles and designing the bedroom in a way that minimizes the risk of falls or other physical harm.

Somnolence

Somnolence refers to a state of abnormal sleepiness or an unusual need for sleep during the day. In psychotherapy and medicine, somnolence is not limited to the feeling of tiredness, but also involves reduced alertness and slowed mental and physical responsiveness. These symptoms can significantly impair the quality of life.

Physiologically, somnolence refers to a kind of intermediate stage between wakefulness and sleep. The affected person can be woken up for a short time by external stimulation, such as speech or touch, but quickly falls back into a dozing state without additional stimulus. This distinguishes somnolence from deeper stages of the decline in consciousness, such as coma or sopor, where wakefulness is only possible through strong stimuli or no longer possible at all.

Psychologically, somnolence can have various causes. In addition to sleep disorders such as sleep apnea or narcolepsy, these also include mental illnesses such as depression, which are often accompanied by persistent fatigue. Drug side effects, especially psychotropic drugs, can also cause somnolence. In addition, it can be a symptom of organic diseases, such as hypothyroidism, chronic fatigue syndrome or diabetes.

In therapy, it is important to clarify the cause of somnolence in order to be able to take the appropriate therapeutic measures. This may include adjusting medication, treating the underlying condition, or specific intervention-related measures, such as chronotherapy to regulate the sleep-wake cycle. Cognitive behavioral therapy (CBT) can also help by altering behaviors and thought patterns that increase fatigue.

For those affected, somnolence often represents a considerable burden in everyday life. It can limit the ability to concentrate and perform and thus impair professional and social activities.

Sopor

Sopor describes a pathological state of deep unconsciousness in which the affected person can only react to strong stimuli, such as pain. This condition is more severe than lightheadedness or somnolence, but not as profound as a coma. In this state, the ability to wake up spontaneously is severely limited, and the sufferer does not show any reactions to verbal or light tactile stimuli.

In clinical practice, Sopor can have various causes, including neurological diseases, severe head injuries, metabolic disorders, poisoning or the effect of certain medications. Psychogenic factors such as extreme psychological stress or traumatic experiences can also lead to a soporous state. Diagnosis requires a careful medical history and a thorough physical and neurological examination. Imaging procedures such as CT or MRI as well as laboratory tests may be necessary to clarify the causes of the condition.

Symptomatically, a patient in the Sopor does not show normal patterns of eye movements or speech. Reflexes may be present but are often diminished or abnormal. When the patient reacts to pain stimuli, this often happens in an uncoordinated and inadequate manner. Vegetative functions such as breathing and circulation are usually preserved, but close monitoring is necessary as complications can occur.

Treatment for Sopor depends on the underlying disease or trigger. In acute cases, emergency medical care may be necessary to protect the patient's life and prevent possible deterioration. This includes measures such as securing the airways, stabilizing the circulation and, if necessary, initiating intensive medical therapy.

Sopor plays a special role in psychotherapy, as the underlying psychological problem must be treated as soon as the patient has returned from the soporous state. This often involves processing trauma or treating mental disorders that may have contributed to the development of the sopor syndrome. Interdisciplinary cooperation with neurologists, internists and other specialists is crucial to ensure comprehensive and long-term effective therapy.

Another word about the prognosis: This varies greatly depending on the cause and the speed with which adequate treatment is initiated. While some patients may recover fully after successful treatment, others are at risk of permanent neurological damage or psychological impairment. Long-term follow-up care and, if necessary, rehabilitative therapy are therefore very important.

Stereotypical movement disorder

Stereotypic movement disorder is a neuropsychiatric disorder characterized by repetitive, involuntary movement patterns that follow a predefined pattern and often occur over a longer period of time. These movements are often rhythmic and can take both simple and more complex forms.

Typical manifestations of the stereotypes include hand fluttering, shaking of the head, turning the body, seesawing or more complex motor sequences such as turning or moving objects. In children, movements such as thumb sucking, hair pulling or biting activities are often seen. Such movements can occur independently of the environment or current activities and are most often not related to specific external stimuli.

Stereotypical movement disorders often occur in early childhood and can be seen in a variety of conditions and developmental disorders. They are often seen in children with autism spectrum disorders (ASD), intellectual disabilities, or other neurodevelopment-related disorders. Genetic diseases such as Rett syndrome or fragile X syndrome also often exhibit stereotypical movements.

The exact cause of stereotypical movement disorder is still not fully understood, but neurobiological factors, including specific dysfunctions in certain brain regions such as the basal ganglia, are thought to play a central role. Environmental factors and genetic predispositions can also influence the manifestation and severity of the disorder.

The impact on daily life can vary significantly. While some patients are barely affected by their stereotypical movements, others may experience serious physical injury or social stigma and isolation. These include skin injuries caused by repeated hitting or scratching, tooth damage from chewing or biting, and problems in the social environment due to the conspicuous behavior.

The diagnosis of the disorder is carried out by means of a comprehensive clinical evaluation, which includes a detailed medical history and observation of specific movement patterns. Differential diagnostics are also important here in order to rule out other diseases such as obsessive-compulsive disorder, tics or sensory impairments.

Therapeutically, a multimodal approach usually shows the best success. Behavioral therapy interventions can help reduce the frequency of movements and improve behavioral control. In addition, special pedagogical approaches and parental and family counselling can have a supportive effect.

In some cases, the use of medications, such as atypical neuroleptics or SSRIs (selective serotonin reuptake inhibitors), may be considered, especially if the symptoms are severe or other therapies do not have sufficient effect.

Stress

Stress refers to a state of physical and/or emotional tension that arises in response to certain internal or external demands. This concept is of great importance in both psychotherapy and general health science, as it has far-reaching implications for human well-being.

Physiological dimensions

From a physiological point of view, stress activates the autonomic nervous system as well as the hypothalamic-pituitary-adrenocortical axis (HPA axis). This leads to the release of hormones such as adrenaline and cortisol. While adrenaline increases the body's alertness in the short term—heart rate, blood pressure, and respiratory rate increase—longer-acting cortisol has more diverse effects, including suppressing the immune system and influencing metabolism.

Psychological dimensions

Psychologically, stress can be triggered by any situation that is perceived as overwhelming, threatening or unpleasant. These can be acute events such as the loss of a loved one or chronic stressors such as persistent job insecurity. An important aspect is the subjective evaluation of the situation, i.e. whether a person perceives it as a stressor or classifies it as manageable.

Emotional and behavioral dimensions

Emotional responses to stress can range from fear and anger to sadness and helplessness. Behaviorally, changes such as increased irritability, social withdrawal, increased or decreased food intake and sleep disorders can occur. Some people also resort to maladaptive coping strategies such as substance abuse or excessive television.

Effects on health

Uncontrolled or chronic stress can lead to various health problems, including cardiovascular disease, gastrointestinal problems, sleep disorders, and mental illnesses such as depression and anxiety disorders. Understanding the potential long-term effects of stress is therefore essential for preventive measures and therapeutic interventions.

Coping

Psychotherapy teaches various approaches to stress management. These include cognitive restructuring to change dysfunctional thought patterns, learning relaxation techniques such as progressive muscle relaxation or mindfulness, and promoting a healthy lifestyle that includes adequate physical activity and a balanced diet. Social support and communication skills also play an important role in reducing and managing stress.

Therapeutic relevance

For the practice of psychotherapy, a well-founded understanding of stress is crucial. Stress can not only be a symptom of mental disorders, but also a triggering and perpetuating factor of them. Therefore, it is important to correctly diagnose stress and treat it effectively, taking a holistic approach that takes into account both physiological and psychological components.

Through the targeted management of stress, clients can significantly gain quality of life, become more resilient and achieve higher levels of emotional and physical well-being.

Stress management training

Stress management training is a structured therapeutic approach to support individuals suffering from increased or chronic stress. The aim of this training is to provide those affected with techniques and strategies that help them to deal with stressful situations more constructively and to minimise the negative effects of stress on their mental and physical health.

At its core, stress management training aims to strengthen the individual self-regulation system. This is achieved through a combination of educational, cognitive, behavioral and relaxation techniques. Educational components include understanding the biological and psychological mechanisms of stress, including physical responses such as the activation of the hypothalamic-pituitary-adrenocortical axis and the release of stress hormones such as cortisol and adrenaline.

An important part of stress management training is cognitive restructuring. In the process, the participants learn to recognize stressful thought patterns and replace them with more beneficial ways of thinking. This process can be supported by techniques such as keeping a thought log, in which stress-inducing situations and the thoughts and feelings associated with them are documented. Intensive reflection and discussion of these protocols help to identify and neutralize cognitive distortions such as black-and-white thinking or catastrophizing.

Behavioral interventions are also central to stress management training. This includes time management techniques, prioritization, and problem-solving strategies. These methods aim to actively change or better cope with stress-causing circumstances. Participants practice in role-plays and through tasks how to apply learned behaviors in real-life situations to expand their scope of action and increase control over stressful situations.

Another important aspect of the training is the teaching of relaxation techniques. Progressive muscle relaxation, autogenic training, mindfulness exercises, and breathing techniques are examples of practices that promote physiological stress reduction. These techniques help activate the body's resting state and reduce the excessive activation of the sympathetic nervous system that typically accompanies stress.

In addition, stress management training can include psychosocial components, such as building and maintaining supportive social networks. In group formats, participants benefit from sharing their experiences and from the support of others who are overcoming similar challenges.

Ultimately, stress management training aims to increase participants' stress resilience, which allows them to better manage future stressful situations. Not only does it promote well-being, but it can also reduce the long-term risks of stress-related health problems such as cardiovascular disease, depression, and anxiety disorders.

Stress reaction

A stress response is the body's and mind's response to perceived threats or demands. It serves as a key mechanism in the human survival system and can be understood as a physical, emotional, cognitive and behavioral response.

On a physical level, the stress response is activated by the so-called "fight-or-flight" system, which is controlled by the sympathetic nervous system. In immediate threatening situations, the body releases adrenaline and norepinephrine, which leads to a fast heart rate, increased blood pressure and rapid breathing. These physiological changes prepare the body for a rapid response. In prolonged stressful situations, the hormone cortisol can also be released, which leads to further physical adaptations.

Emotionally, stress can trigger various feelings, including fear, anger, frustration, or overwhelm. These emotions often serve to focus attention and motivate energetic actions. However, with prolonged stress, they can lead to emotional exhaustion and even serious mental states such as anxiety disorders or depression.

Cognitively, stress manifests itself through a change in mindset and perception. Sufferers may have difficulty thinking clearly, making decisions, or concentrating. A so-called tunnel perception often occurs, in which the focus is exclusively on the stress-triggering situation. Long-term stress can impair memory and increase the risk of cognitive impairment.

In terms of behavior, stress can cause different reactions, most of which are aimed at coping with or avoiding the threat. These behaviors can take adaptive forms, such as developing coping strategies or seeking social support. However, they can also express themselves maladaptively, e.g. through aggressive behaviour, social withdrawal, excessive consumption of alcohol or drugs or compulsive behaviour.

The stress response is closely linked to the individual coping style and personal resources. While short-term, acute stress can play a protective and performance-enhancing role, chronic stress poses significant health risks, both physically and psychologically.

In psychotherapeutic practice, understanding the stress response is essential, as many mental disorders are either caused or exacerbated by chronic stress. Corresponding interventions aim to identify the stress triggers, modify stress processing and promote adaptive stress management strategies. Methods such as cognitive behavioral therapy (CBT), mindfulness-based stress reduction (MBSR) or mindfulness-based approaches can be helpful here.

Stupor

Stupor is a clinical symptom characterized by a state of deep clouding of consciousness in which the affected person responds little or not at all to external stimuli. This condition can be both psychological and neurological and represents a serious impairment in daily life.

In psychotherapy, stupor is often observed in connection with severe affective disorders such as catatonic schizophrenia, severe depression or traumatic experiences. In a stuporous state, those affected show a considerable reduction in motor activity up to complete immobility. Although the person's sensorium is mostly intact, they do not appear to be able to respond to environmental stimuli or perform self-initiated movements.

A central feature of the stupors is the rigid posture called waxy flexibility, in which the limbs and body remain in an unusual position when they are moved by another person. This suggests that muscle tension has a not inconsiderable degree of stiffness. At the same time, there may be accompanying symptoms such as reduced speech production (mutism) and sometimes catatonic features in which the patient performs stereotypical movements.

In differential diagnosis, it is important to distinguish stupor from conditions such as coma, deep sleep or drug-induced loss of consciousness. The diagnostic distinction is made by a detailed anamnesis and physical examination. This specifically looks for psychiatric, neurological and medical causes that could cause a stuporous state.

Therapeutically, dealing with stupor is challenging. In the case of psychogenic causes, drug treatment with antidepressants, antipsychotics or benzodiazepines may be necessary. In addition, the condition requires intensive psychotherapeutic and nursing care. In the therapeutic setting, cognitive-behavioral therapeutic approaches or supportive measures such as creative forms of therapy can make a valuable contribution to treatment.

Suicidal tendencies according to Pöldinger

The suicidal phases according to Pöldinger serve as a model description of the development and dynamics of suicidal crises. This concept divides the course of suicidal thoughts and actions into three phases, which results in a better understanding of the escalation of such crises and allows preventive measures to be applied in a targeted manner.

Recital 1 (Consideration)

In the first phase, those affected deal with the idea of suicide, but without making concrete plans. This period can be characterized by persistent despair, hopelessness and inner emptiness. The person begins to think about his or her life situation and to look for alternative ways out. At the same time, there is often a lack of firm determination in this phase, the thoughts remain fleeting and theoretical. Talking about their thoughts can be difficult at this stage, as they feel ashamed of their thoughts or feel that no one understands them. A deep feeling of loneliness often pervades the consideration phase.

2. Ambivalence phase (ambivalence)

The second phase is characterized by an intense inner conflict. The people fluctuate between the desire to live and the need to end their lives. Here, a concrete examination of different methods and possibilities of suicide develops, but there is still a clear ambivalence, which manifests itself, for example, in the hope that an intervention from outside will take place or that their living conditions will improve. Often, those affected signal this ambivalence through hints in conversations or changes in behavior, which can often be understood as cries for help. In this phase, it is elementary to listen empathetically and to take hidden clues seriously.

3. Decision phase (decision)

In the last phase, the affected person has made a clear decision to commit suicide and often feels a paradoxical calm and relief. The ambivalence gives way to increased determination, so that the affected person makes concrete preparations, such as collecting funds or providing suicide tools. This phase can be characterized by sudden mood lifts or rational, almost emotionless behavior, as the person considers their burden resolved. According to this change, they can organize their affairs, write farewell letters or contact people with whom they want to conclude. A potentially life-saving intervention requires quick and decisive action through a stable network of relatives, friends and professionals.

Pöldinger's model is valuable for the diagnosis and prevention of suicides in therapeutic practice. It enables therapists to detect suicidal processes at an early stage and to develop targeted prevention strategies. Understanding these phases supports both direct intervention and long-term follow-up of people at risk of suicide.

Suicide

Suicide represents the deliberate and independent act of a person to end their own life. This phenomenon is extremely complex and multi-layered and can have various triggering factors, including mental illness, personal crises, social isolation or persistent suffering.

In psychotherapy, suicide is understood not only as a symptom of an underlying mental or emotional disorder, but also as a response to a feeling of overwhelming hopelessness and hopelessness. People who are suicidal often feel that death is the only way to escape their suffering. This can be due to severe depression, anxiety disorders, severe trauma, or other mental illnesses such as schizophrenia or bipolar disorder. Substance abuse can also increase suicidal thoughts and actions.

A central aspect in the treatment of suicidal patients is to assess the risk of suicide and to take appropriate intervention measures. This includes recording suicidal thoughts, plans, and existing suicide attempts, as well as assessing the severity and urgency of the suicidal crisis. Close monitoring and the development of a safety plan are crucial steps in the therapeutic process to minimize the risk of suicide.

Therapists often work with different therapeutic approaches and techniques to address suicidal thoughts and behaviors. These include cognitive behavioral therapy (CBT), dialectical behavioral therapy (DBT), and other evidence-based methods. These approaches aim to change dysfunctional thought patterns, develop coping strategies, and strengthen social support systems.

In acute cases, inpatient treatment may be necessary to ensure the safety of the patient. Psychotropic drugs can also be used, especially if there is an underlying psychiatric disorder such as severe depression. Close follow-up care and long-term psychotherapeutic support are crucial to prevent relapses and enable the patient to develop healthier life strategies.

Dealing with the topic of suicide in psychotherapy requires a high degree of sensitivity, empathy and professional competence from therapists. Therapists must be able to create a safe and supportive environment where patients can talk openly about their feelings and thoughts without fear of stigma or judgment.

In addition, suicide prevention also includes working with the social environment of the affected person in order to promote support and understanding. Education and training for family members and friends can help to identify warning signs early on and respond appropriately.

Suicide is a serious issue in psychotherapeutic practice that requires a deep understanding of the underlying factors and comprehensive, compassionate care. Continuous research and education in this field are essential to ensure the best possible support and treatment for suicidal patients.

Supervision

Supervision is a methodically guided reflection and counselling process that has been specially developed for professionals in psychosocial professions. In psychotherapy, supervision plays a central role in ensuring the quality of therapeutic work and promoting the professional development of therapists.

The core of supervision is the offer of a safe space in which therapists can discuss their professional experiences and challenges. The supervisor, usually an experienced therapist or a proven expert in the field, leads this process. Through targeted questions, feedback and professional impulses, the supervisor helps the therapist to gain new perspectives on his work and to expand his possibilities for action.

Supervision encompasses various dimensions: the reflection of the therapeutic relationship, the processing of case histories, the examination of one's own emotional reactions and the clarification of professional roles. It can take place in individual as well as in group settings, whereby in group supervisions the exchange among colleagues can have additional enriching effects.

An essential aspect of supervision is the promotion of self-reflection. Therapists are encouraged to recognize and understand their own transference and countertransference processes. This helps to clarify the therapeutic relationship and to uncover possible blind spots in one's own actions. In addition, emotional relief plays an important role, as working with suffering people can also lead to emotional stress for therapists.

On the practical level, supervision also supports the structuring and planning of the therapy processes. By exploring and discussing specific case studies, new therapeutic interventions can be tested and the effectiveness of existing methods can be questioned.

In addition, supervision can also concern organizational and institutional issues. Questions of cooperation in the team, dealing with institutional requirements or ethical issues are typical topics that are addressed in supervision.

Supervisor/Supervisor

In psychotherapy, care or the role of a caregiver is understood to be comprehensive and continuous support of a person by a professional or a relative in the field of mental health. Care encompasses a range of activities and responsibilities that focus on the well-being and health of the client.

A caregiver can work both formally and informally. Formal caregivers are often professional therapists, social workers or caregivers who are specially trained and legitimized by professional qualifications to support mentally stressed people. Informal caregivers, on the other hand, are often family members or friends who care about the mental and emotional health of the person concerned.

The care process often begins with a detailed diagnosis in order to identify the exact psychological problem of the client. On the basis of this diagnosis, the caregiver works with the client to develop individual therapy goals and methods. The caregiver plays a central role as a companion, supporter and mediator.

Caregivers act as a link between the client and the various psychosocial and medical resources available. They coordinate appointments, advise on various therapy options and facilitate access to medication, therapy groups or other supportive measures.

A crucial point of care is emotional support. Caregivers offer an open ear, give the client a feeling of security and acceptance and promote their resilience and self-confidence. Empathy, patience and the ability to build a trusting relationship are essential qualities of a good caregiver.

Aspects that go beyond therapy, such as support with everyday tasks, help with vocational rehabilitation or the mediation of social contacts, can also be part of the care. The aim is to enable the client to lead a self-determined life despite his or her mental impairments.

Caregivers must also undergo continuous training in order to stay up to date with the latest research and therapeutic approaches. This often includes supervision and participation in specialist seminars.

In summary, the role of a caregiver can be described as extremely complex and indispensable. It includes professional support and therapeutic accompaniment as well as personal attention and emotional help, making an indispensable contribution to the stability and improvement of the quality of life of mentally stressed people.

Systemic therapy

Systemic therapy is a psychotherapeutic approach that focuses on the interactions and relationships within a system, be it a family, a couple relationship, a team, or a community. This approach is based on the assumption that human behaviour and psychological problems should not be considered in isolation, but should always be understood in the context of the interactions and relationships of the people involved.

At the heart of systemic therapy is the conviction that every person is part of a network of relationships that significantly influences their attitudes, emotions and behaviors. Rather than focusing only on the individual and their symptoms, Systemic Therapy examines the dynamics and patterns that exist within the system. The aim is to identify the connections and mechanisms that lead to the current difficulties.

A central aspect of systemic therapy is the idea of circularity. This states that cause and effect are always reciprocal in social systems. Instead of looking for linear causal chains – i.e. simple cause-and-effect relationships – the systemic therapist looks at the interactions and feedback loops within the system. This promotes an understanding of how certain behaviors can mutually condition and reinforce each other.

Another fundamental concept is the contextual dependence of human behavior. Systemic therapy recognizes that different contexts can produce different behavioral tendencies. What may seem problematic in one context may be entirely appropriate in another. Therefore, an attempt is made to take into account the different life contexts of the clients and to understand their significance for the respective problem behavior.

In systemic therapy, the therapist often acts as a moderator and less as an expert. It asks questions that encourage the system to recognize its own patterns and develop solutions, rather than giving direct advice or recommendations for action. A well-known method is circular questioning, in which the relationship perspectives within the system are illuminated through targeted questions. This also raises awareness of the perspectives and perceptions of other participants.

A central goal of Systemic Therapy is to promote the autonomy and self-efficacy of the client. The therapeutic process is intended to strengthen the ability to shape one's own relationships and interactions more consciously and to initiate constructive changes in the system. This can be done, for example, by learning new communication and behavioral strategies or by understanding and changing dysfunctional relationship patterns.

Systemic therapists use a variety of methods and techniques that are adapted to the individual needs and situations of the client. These include, among others, genograms that visually represent family structure and dynamics, constellations and sculptures that make symbolic representations of relationships and hierarchies visible in space, as well as narrative techniques that help clients reformulate their own story and discover alternative meanings and possibilities for action.

The effectiveness of systemic therapy has been proven by numerous studies, especially in the work with families and couples. It is used for a variety of psychological and psychosocial problems, including communication disorders, conflicts, addiction, depression, anxiety disorders and psychosomatic illnesses.

Through its holistic and resource-oriented approach, Systemic Therapy offers a flexible and effective way to bring about profound changes in clients' relationships and behavior. The focus is always on understanding the individual in his or her entire living environment, which can lead to sustainable and comprehensive improvements.

Therapeutic Alliance

The therapeutic alliance refers to the cooperative, trusting and empathetic relationship between a therapist and his patient. This connection is one of the central components for the success of psychotherapy and forms the foundation of the therapeutic process. The therapeutic alliance is characterized by several key features that allow for a deep, systematic therapeutic process.

An essential part of the therapeutic alliance is mutual trust. The patient must feel the security and confidence of being able to open up to the therapist without fear of judgment or sanctions. This trust is promoted by consistency, reliability and empathy on the part of the therapist.

Another important aspect is the agreement between therapist and patient regarding the therapy goals and the therapeutic approach. It is essential that both parties develop a common understanding of what is to be achieved in therapy and how these goals can be realized. This agreement leads to the establishment of a coherent and targeted treatment plan.

The emotional bond between therapist and patient also plays an important role. This bond allows the patient to express themselves freely and discuss even difficult or painful topics. The therapist supports this process through active listening, empathy, and understanding, which fosters a deeper emotional connection.

Another vital aspect of the therapeutic alliance is the cooperation and active participation of the patient in the therapeutic process. The patient should feel like an active partner in therapy and not just a passive recipient of interventions. This increases the patient's commitment and motivation, which increases the chances of success of the therapy.

Transparency and openness are equally crucial for the therapeutic alliance. The therapist should always inform the patient about the therapeutic process, the methods used and the progress. This creates clarity and promotes a feeling of co-creation and control in the patient.

Obstacles in the therapeutic alliance can significantly impair the success of therapy. It is the therapist's task to recognize and address any tensions, misunderstandings or resistance at an early stage. Through supervision and reflection, the therapist can continuously evaluate and optimize his relationship with the patient.

Therapeutic limits

Therapeutic boundaries are essential framework conditions that structure and secure the professional relationship between a psychotherapist and his client. These limits serve as protective mechanisms for both parties and ensure effective and ethical therapy.

In a therapeutic context, boundaries define the roles, responsibilities, and emotional interactions between therapist and client. They help to maintain a clear distance, which is indispensable to ensure objectivity and professionalism. Without these boundaries, there could be confusion about the nature of the relationship, which could disrupt the therapeutic balance and healing process.

A central aspect of therapeutic boundaries is the temporal and spatial structure. This includes firmly adhering to session times as well as defining a clear physical space for therapy in which both parties interact. The therapist is responsible for ensuring that these rules are consistently adhered to in order to provide reliable consistency and confidentiality.

Another important component of therapeutic boundaries concerns the emotional and personal bond. The therapist must maintain a professional distance and must not enter into friendships or more intimate relationships with the client. This distance protects the client from potential exploitation and the therapist from role conflicts and emotional overload.

Communication within therapy is also strictly regulated. The therapist shares professional insights, but avoids revealing personal information about himself so as not to unnecessarily influence the dynamics of the therapist-client relationship. This helps the client to focus solely on their own process and healing.

Restrictive rules apply with regard to physical interactions. Physical contact is avoided in most therapeutic settings unless there is a clear therapeutic reason and the boundaries are clearly discussed and established beforehand. This is to prevent misunderstandings and boundary violations that could affect both the therapeutic process and the client's well-being.

Trustworthiness and secrecy are further elementary aspects of therapeutic limits. The therapist is obliged to treat all content discussed in therapy confidentially, unless there is a legal obligation to report it, for example in cases of acute danger to himself or others.

Therapeutic relationship

The therapeutic relationship, also known as the working relationship or therapeutic alliance, is the foundation and one of the central components of the psychotherapeutic process. It refers to the professional, respectful and trusting relationship between therapist and client, which is characterized by mutual understanding and cooperation.

A successful therapeutic relationship is supported by several core factors:

Trust: Trust is the basis of every therapeutic relationship. The client must feel that they can confide in the therapist their most intimate thoughts and feelings without being judged or judged. This trust is built through repeated positive interactions and the therapist's reliability.

Empathy: Empathy on the part of the therapist is crucial. It enables the therapist to understand the client's inner experiences and to develop a deep understanding of their situation. Empathy is manifested in attentive listening, appropriate response to emotional expressions, and the need to understand the client's perspective.

Authenticity: The therapist must be authentic and genuine in their interaction with the client. He should not play an artificial or artificial role, but show his real personality and human qualities. Authenticity promotes trust and honesty in the therapeutic relationship.

Respect and appreciation: Respecting the client as a person with their own rights, wishes and needs is indispensable. Appreciation is shown by taking the client seriously, appreciating his autonomy and preserving his dignity, regardless of his problems or behaviors.

Shared goals: Developing common, well-defined goals is another key factor in an effective therapeutic relationship. The therapist and client work together to set realistic and achievable goals for therapy. These goals should be reviewed regularly and adjusted as needed to ensure progress.

Communication: Open and effective communication is essential. The therapist should speak clearly and intelligibly and at the same time listen attentively. Misunderstandings should be avoided, and if they occur, they should be clarified immediately.

Boundaries and structure: A clearly defined structure and appropriate boundaries within the therapeutic relationship offer the client security and orientation. This includes adherence to agreed meeting times, the confidentiality of the conversations and the conscious handling of one's own role and competencies as a therapist.

Flexibility: The therapist should be able to respond flexibly to the individual needs and uniqueness of the client. This requires adaptability and creativity to adapt the methods and techniques of therapy to the client's changing circumstances and progress.

In summary, the therapeutic relationship forms the framework within which healing and change can happen. It is a dynamic, processual aspect of therapy that must be continuously nurtured and strengthened to ensure positive and effective collaboration.

Therapist's self-care

Therapist self-care describes the personal practice by which psychotherapists maintain their physical, emotional, and mental health in order to provide effective support to their clients. This self-care is particularly essential in a profession that is characterized by intensive emotional work and high psychological stress. Self-care can be divided into different categories, including physical, emotional, social, and professional self-care.

In physical self-care, therapists take care of their bodies through regular exercise, a balanced diet, adequate sleep, and regular health checks. These measures help keep the body healthy and resilient to stress.

Emotional self-care refers to the need to manage one's feelings and emotions in a healthy and constructive way. Therapists are often confronted with the emotional difficulties of their clients and therefore have to develop mechanisms to process these stresses. This can be done through personal therapy, supervision, reflection, and maintaining a stable emotional state. A clear demarcation between work and private life also helps to maintain emotional integrity.

Social self-care involves nurturing relationships outside of the therapeutic context. A strong personal network of family and friends provides emotional support and allows you to relax in a social setting. This social support is crucial to experiencing a sense of belonging and emotional balance.

Professional self-care, on the other hand, refers to measures that affect the professional framework. This includes continuous training, adherence to ethical standards, collegial advice and a well-organised work structure. Not only does this help stay professionally up-to-date, but it also prevents the feeling of isolation that can arise from this often lonely work.

Self-care is not just seen as a one-time goal, but as an ongoing process of self-reflection and adaptation. Successful self-care requires recognizing and acknowledging one's own needs and consciously creating time and space for their fulfillment. Techniques such as time management, keeping diaries or mindfulness exercises can be helpful for this.

A lack of self-care can have serious consequences, such as burnout, empathy fatigue, and a reduced ability to work effectively. The ability to take care of oneself and to treat oneself well is directly reflected in the quality of therapeutic work. A healthy, balanced life is therefore the basis for long-term fulfillment and effectiveness in psychotherapy.

Therapy goals

Therapy goals are specific, often measurable results that both the client and the therapist formulate at the beginning of therapy. These goals serve as a guide for the therapeutic process, provide orientation and make it possible to evaluate progress in the course of therapy.

Therapy goals are developed in close cooperation between therapist and client. They should be realistic, achievable, and individually tailored to the client's needs and resources. An effective therapy conversation helps to define clear goals by clarifying the current difficulties that the client is experiencing, as well as their wishes and expectations for therapy.

An essential feature of therapy goals is their concretization. Instead of formulating general concerns such as "I want to feel better", a concrete goal will be, for example: "I want to learn to cope better with my anxiety attacks so that I can go back to work regularly." This specification makes it easier to measure the success of the therapy and to visualize the client's progress.

The formulation of therapy goals encompasses various dimensions, including emotional, cognitive, behavioral and interpersonal areas. A client with depression might have emotional goals, such as reducing sadness, cognitive goals, such as changing negative thought patterns, and behavioral goals, such as increasing social activity.

In addition, therapy goals should be flexible and dynamic. Since the therapeutic process often involves unpredictable developments, it makes sense to regularly review and adjust the goals. This review makes it possible to incorporate new insights and advances and ensure that therapy continues to be aligned with the client's needs.

The type and scope of the therapy goals can differ depending on the therapeutic approach and the respective problem of the client. In cognitive behavioral therapy, for example, the goals could be very specific and behavioral, while in humanistic therapy, the focus is more on general personal development and self-actualization.

Last but not least, therapy goals provide a motivating structure for both the client and the therapist. For the client, achievable intermediate goals create a sense of achievement that strengthens self-confidence and maintains motivation. For the therapist, clearly defined goals provide a systematic framework for planning and conducting the therapeutic sessions.

Thinking disorders

Thinking disorders, an important field within psychopathology, refer to qualitative and quantitative impairments of the thought process. These disorders can have different dimensions and expressions that affect an individual's thinking in different ways. They often manifest themselves in the form of confusion, leaps of thought, fixation on certain topics or the inability to think logically and coherently. Thinking disorders can occur in both form and content, with formal thinking disorders affecting the structure and flow of thought, and substantive thinking disorders affecting the thoughts themselves.

Formal thinking disorders affect the way thoughts are ordered and expressed. Examples are:

- **Mind flight (mind hunt):** Here, the person experiences accelerated thinking with rapid transitions between thoughts. This can lead to incoherent or only loosely connected statements.
- **Mind Breaking**: The flow of thoughts is suddenly interrupted, and the person loses the thread of the conversation, resulting in an abrupt pause in communication.
- **Erratic thinking**: Thoughts move in leaps and bounds between different, often unrelated, topics, resulting in a disjointed conversation.
- **Perseveration**: Here, the person repeats the same thoughts or words over and over again, regardless of context or relevance.

Content-related thinking disorders include abnormal thought content and beliefs. These include:

- **Delusions**: Firm, irrational beliefs that are maintained despite evidence to the contrary. These can take various forms, such as paranoia, megalomania or relationship delusions.
- **Obsessive thoughts**: Intrusive, intrusive thoughts that seem inappropriate or distressing to the person, and are often associated with compulsions to neutralize these thoughts.
- **Overvalued ideas**: Highly overrated thoughts that dominate the person's thoughts and actions, often without the rigid characteristics of delusion.

Thinking disorders can occur in a variety of mental illnesses, including schizophrenia, mood disorders, anxiety disorders, and neurological conditions such as dementia. The impact on daily life is significant, as it affects rational thinking, decision-making, and communication skills.

The diagnosis of thinking disorders requires careful observation and questioning by trained professionals. It is essential to recognize the difference between culturally accepted beliefs and pathological thought disorders in order to make an accurate diagnosis. Therapeutic approaches may include drug treatments, psychotherapeutic interventions, or a combination of both, depending on the underlying cause and severity of the disorder.

Tick disorders

Tic disorders are neuropsychiatric disorders that manifest themselves through involuntary, sudden, rapid, repetitive and non-rhythmic movements or vocalizations. These tics can be motor or vocal in nature and vary in frequency and intensity, can include simple movements such as blinking, shaking the head or grimacing, or more complex actions such as jumping, tapping or repeating certain movements.

An essential category of tic disorders is Tourette's syndrome, in which both multiple motor and at least one vocal tic must exist over a period of more than one year. Other categories include transient, chronic motor or vocal tic disorders, in which either motor or vocal tics are present and which persist for different periods of time.

Symptoms usually begin in childhood, often between the ages of four and six, and reach their peak in early adolescence, although the intensity often decreases in adulthood. The exact causes of tic disorders are complex and multifactorial, and include genetic predispositions, neurobiological factors, and environmental factors. Studies suggest that dysfunctions in the basal ganglia, a brain region that regulates movements, may play a central role.

From a psychotherapeutic point of view, it is important to record the severity of the tics and the resulting impairment in different areas of life. Differentiated diagnostics play an essential role in ruling out other neurological or psychological diseases. Behavioral therapy approaches are often used for therapy, such as habit reversal training, which aims to increase awareness of the tics and train alternative behaviors that reduce the likelihood of the tics occurring.

In addition to behavioral therapy, drug approaches can also be considered, especially in the case of severe symptoms or if there is a severe functional impairment. Various medications are used for this purpose, such as neuroleptics or centrally active substances.

In addition to the core symptoms of tics, those affected can also often experience comorbid disorders such as attention deficit/hyperactivity disorder (ADHD), obsessive-compulsive disorder, anxiety disorders or depression. Treatment should therefore be comprehensively designed to adequately address these comorbidities and improve patients' quality of life.

Transactional analysis

Transactional analysis (TA) is a psychotherapeutic and counseling method developed by Eric Berne in the 1950s. It is based on the assumption that human behavior is due to previous experiences and the resulting internal psychological states. Transactional analysis is a comprehensive model that deals with communication and personality structure, interpersonal relationships and self-perception within psychological structures, among other things.

The basic unit of transactional analysis is "transactions", which consist of a stimulus and a reaction. Each transaction involves at least two people, and each person can act from three different ego states: the parent ego, the adult ego and the child ego.

1. **Parent-ego**: This state consists of behaviors, feelings, and attitudes that have been inherited from the parents or parental figures. It is divided into the critical parent ego, which can be judgmental, moralizing or punishing, and the caring parent ego, which shows supportive and nurturing behavior.
2. **Adult ego**: In this state, a person acts rationally, objectively and appropriately for the situation. The adult ego state is the one that acts on the basis of current reality and not on the basis of past experiences or emotional reactions. He is characterized by a factual and analytical approach.
3. **Child-ego**: This state reflects the behaviors, feelings and attitudes that originate from one's own childhood. The child ego can be divided into the natural child ego, which represents free, spontaneous behavior focused on immediate needs, and the adapted child ego, which is characterized by obedience and subordination.

The analysis of these ego states helps therapists and clients to understand from which internalized state a person reacts in certain situations and enables the targeted promotion of healthy interactions.

Another central concept of transactional analysis is the "life script theory". A life script is an unconscious life plan that is often formed in childhood and strengthened by repeated interactions and decisions across the lifespan. This plan has a significant influence on how an individual shapes his or her life and what successes or failures he or she experiences. The therapeutic process aims to identify and modify dysfunctional scripts and to enable clients to act freely and self-determinedly.

Transactional analysis also makes use of concepts from the field of game theory and levels of conflict. So-called "games" are described as recurring and manipulative patterns of behavior that serve to fulfill unconscious needs. These games often follow a predictable course and usually end in a negative emotional experience, although those involved do not always consciously realize this.

In the therapeutic work with transactional analysis, interventions are developed to help clients to make their transactions more conscious and constructive, to break dysfunctional communication patterns, to promote healthy and authentic relationships and to increase autonomy, awareness and spontaneity.

Transfer

Transference is a central concept in psychotherapy, especially within the psychoanalytic and psychodynamic approaches. This is the unconscious relocation of feelings, desires, expectations and behavioural patterns that were originally developed in previous relationships – usually with important attachment figures such as parents or siblings – to the therapist. These processes often happen unconsciously, so that the client initially has no conscious control over them.

In the therapeutic setting, transmission can take a variety of forms. For example, a client might transfer feelings of admiration, dependence, or love that originally existed toward a parent to the therapist. Likewise, negative emotions such as mistrust, anger or disappointment can occur that result from similar previous experiences. The relationship between client and therapist is thus influenced in a complex way and makes it possible to recognize and work on deeply hidden emotional patterns and conflicts from childhood.

Transference is a powerful diagnostic and therapeutic tool because it reveals the client's emotional dynamics and inner conflicts. The therapist can observe and analyze these processes in order to gain a deeper understanding of the client's psychological structure. This dynamic can then be used in therapy to help the client identify and change patterns that are no longer helpful and often destructive in the present life.

An essential part of working with transference is to carefully address it and make the client aware of it without overwhelming him or devaluing his feelings and reactions. This requires a high level of sensitivity and professional competence on the part of the therapist. Successful work with transference can lead to a profound change in the client's personality and emotional life, as it helps heal old wounds and establish new, healthier relationship patterns.

Trauma therapy

Trauma therapy refers to a specialized area of psychotherapy that is dedicated to the treatment of post-traumatic stress disorders. These can be different types of trauma, such as sexual, physical or emotional abuse, natural disasters, accidents or even war-related experiences. Trauma therapy is designed to help those affected to process traumatic experiences and alleviate the resulting psychological suffering.

An important part of trauma therapy is the creation of a safe therapeutic framework in which the patient can gain confidence and open up. Security and stability are basic prerequisites for the successful processing of traumatic experiences. The therapist must act sensitively, patiently and without prejudice in order to convey a feeling of security and understanding.

Various therapeutic methods are used in trauma therapy, each of which depends on the type and severity of the trauma and the individual needs of the patient. A widely used method is EMDR (Eye Movement Desensitization and Reprocessing), in which the processing of traumatic memories is supported by targeted eye movements and stimulation. This method can help mitigate the intense emotional responses to the trauma.

Cognitive behavioral therapy (CBT) also plays a central role in trauma therapy. It helps patients to recognize and change dysfunctional thought patterns. By dealing with the altered memory content and beliefs, the patient learns to place the events experienced in a different, less stressful context.

Narrative exposure therapy (NET) is another proven method, especially in patients with complex trauma. Here, the patient's life story is worked through in detail in a safe therapeutic setting. This method aims to develop a coherent narrative that allows stressful experiences to be placed in a broader life context.

In addition to these techniques, mindfulness-based stress reduction (MBST) and dialectical behavioral therapy (DBT) are often used to promote emotional regulation and resilience. These methods help patients deal with stress, anxiety, and other anxiety that can be triggered by traumatic experiences.

Another important aspect is working with body-oriented procedures, such as Somatic Experiencing and trauma-focused forms of body therapy. These approaches emphasize the connection between body and mind and help patients alleviate the physical manifestations of trauma.

The effectiveness of trauma therapy depends decisively on the individual adaptation of the treatment to the respective patient. Each person reacts differently to trauma and requires a tailor-made therapeutic approach. The success of trauma therapy is often reflected in the improvement of everyday life, the reduction of symptoms of post-traumatic stress disorder and the restoration of a sense of control and autonomy in the life of the affected person.

Treatment

A treatment plan is a central part of psychotherapeutic work and represents a structured and systematic approach to effectively address a patient's psychological problems and needs. It acts as a guideline that guides the therapeutic process and provides guidance and clarity to both the therapist and the patient.

A treatment plan usually begins with a comprehensive diagnostic phase, during which the therapist takes a thorough medical history, makes diagnoses, and identifies the patient's main problems as well as potential risk factors. This is done through interviews, standardized questionnaires, behavioral observations and, if necessary, physical examinations. The findings from this diagnostic phase form the basis for the formulation of concrete therapy goals.

The therapy goals are specific, measurable, achievable, relevant and time-bound (SMART) goals that are individually tailored to the patient. These goals can be divided into short-term and long-term goals. Short-term goals are often designed to alleviate immediate symptoms, while long-term goals seek deeper and more lasting changes, such as improving interpersonal relationships or increasing resilience.

A treatment plan also includes the selection of therapeutic interventions and methods to be used to achieve the defined goals. Depending on the disorder, patient preference and theoretical approach of the therapist, various psychotherapeutic techniques such as cognitive behavioral therapy, psychodynamic therapy, systemic therapy or humanistic approaches are taken into account. A well-designed treatment plan should be flexible and allow room for adjustment, as the therapeutic process is dynamic and must respond to changes in the patient's condition and needs.

The determination of the frequency and duration of sessions as well as the estimation of an expected duration of therapy are also essential components of the treatment plan. These organizational aspects help to define the framework of therapy and ensure that there is enough time and space to work on the problems.

An important part of the treatment plan is the regular review and evaluation of the progress of therapy. The therapist continuously evaluates whether the set goals are being achieved and whether the methods used are effective. If necessary, adjustments are made to optimize the therapy process. These evaluation phases promote both transparency and the joint responsibility of therapist and patient for the success of the therapy.

In addition, if necessary, the treatment plan also includes the involvement of other professionals or referrals to additional resources such as psychosocial services, medical care or support groups. The interdisciplinary cooperation ensures that the patient receives holistic support.

Finally, the treatment plan also includes a final phase in which the success of therapy is consolidated and strategies for relapse prevention are developed. The goal of this phase is to enable the patient to independently apply the strategies and skills they have learned in everyday life and thus maintain long-term improvements.

Treatment contract

A treatment contract forms the legal basis for the therapeutic relationship between the psychotherapist and the patient. It describes in detail the rights and obligations of both parties and ensures that there is clarity and transparency about the essential aspects of the therapy.

Such a contract usually contains several central elements. First, it describes the type of therapy planned, including the methods and techniques used by the therapist. This can include various psychotherapeutic approaches such as cognitive behavioral therapy, depth psychology-based psychotherapy or systemic therapy.

Furthermore, the treatment contract addresses organizational details such as the frequency and duration of the sessions, the location of the meeting, as well as the costs and billing modalities. This also includes regulations on cancellation fees for appointments that are not cancelled in time and how to deal with delays.

A particularly important component is the duty of confidentiality, which ensures that all content discussed in the course of therapy is treated confidentially. Exceptions to this rule are only made in legally defined cases, for example if there is acute danger to oneself or others or if certain reportable crimes become known.

Questions of consent to therapy, information about possible risks and side effects as well as the limits of therapy are also set out in the contract. This includes the patient's right to discontinue therapy at any time and the therapist's right to terminate treatment under certain circumstances, such as if a relationship of trust cannot be established.

Another component can be dealing with emergencies and crisis situations, including information about how and when the therapist can be reached outside of regular sessions.

Finally, the treatment contract often refers to the possibility and conditions for supervision or the involvement of other specialists, especially in the case of complex or lengthy therapeutic processes.

The treatment contract not only serves to protect the legal interests of both parties, but also promotes clear and structured communication and creates a secure basis for the therapeutic process.

Unconsciousness

Disorders of consciousness are impairments of the normal state of consciousness that can manifest themselves in various areas of experience and behavior. These disorders affect both the quantitative and the qualitative dimensions of consciousness. Quantitative disorders of consciousness range from lightheadedness to somnolence to coma, although the intensity and depth of these states can vary.

Quantitative disorders of consciousness are often characterized by reduced alertness and attention. A patient with drowsiness, for example, shows a significant slowdown in his thoughts and actions, whereas a somnolent patient is difficult to awaken by external stimuli. Patients in a coma are no longer responsive and show no reactions to external influences.

Qualitative disorders of consciousness, on the other hand, describe changes in the clarity and structure of consciousness. These include phenomena such as narrowing of consciousness, shift in consciousness and expansion of consciousness. A narrowing of consciousness is manifested by a clear limitation of the range of experience and perception. The affected person is strongly focused on a specific experience or action, while the perception of the environment is severely limited.

Shifts in consciousness often involve a change in the subjective experience of space, time and one's own person. These shifts can manifest themselves in states such as depersonalization and derealization, in which one's self and environment are perceived as alien or unreal.

Expansions of consciousness often include an increased sense of oneness with the environment or transcendent experiences. Such changes often occur in the context of therapeutic processes, meditation, or under the influence of psychedelic substances.

Causes of disorders of consciousness can be diverse and range from neurological and psychiatric diseases to intoxications and metabolic and systemic disorders. Diagnostics and therapy therefore require an interdisciplinary approach that includes careful anamnesis, neurological examinations and, if necessary, imaging procedures.

The therapeutic approach is highly dependent on the underlying cause of the disturbance of consciousness. For example, somatic causes such as brain injury, inflammation or intoxication may require specialized medical interventions, while psychological causes such as dissociative disorders or acute psychotic episodes require psychotherapeutic treatment and possibly psychiatric medication.

Vulnerability

In psychotherapy, vulnerability refers to the susceptibility or sensitivity of an individual to psychological stress and stressors. This sensitivity can manifest itself in different circumstances and is often due to a combination of genetic, biological, psychological and social factors.

At the genetic and biological level, vulnerability can be caused by a family history of certain mental disorders. For example, an increased sensitivity of the neurobiological stress system, i.e. the hypothalamic-pituitary-adrenocortical axis (HPA axis), can lead to an increased probability of psychologically decompensating in stressful situations. Neurotransmitter imbalances and neuronal structures that cause an increased willingness to react to stress signals also play a role.

Psychologically, vulnerability includes aspects of personality structure and previous life experiences. Individuals with low self-esteem, inadequate coping strategies, and traumatic childhood experiences are at higher risk of developing mental health problems. The individual's ability to regulate emotions and manage stress is a central factor. People with pronounced vulnerability tend to experience challenges and conflicts as overwhelming and, conversely, underestimate their ability to deal with them effectively.

At the social level, vulnerability can be influenced by the quality and quantity of social support. A stable and strong social network can act as a protective factor. Lack of social resources, isolation and hostile or excessive stress in the social environment, on the other hand, can increase sensitivity to mental disorders. Critical life events such as the loss of a loved one or job-related stress are of particular importance.

Feedback on this book

The satisfaction of our readers is important to us, and we would be very happy if you could send us your feedback on the book.

We would like to ask you to take a moment to write a customer review on Amazon. In this way, you support other readers in making purchasing decisions and contribute to constantly improving our offer.

Thank you very much!

IMPRESSUM
Information according to § 5 TMG:
Markus Gohlke
c/o IP-Management #16265
Ludwig-Erhard-Str. 18
20459 Hamburg
Contact:
E-mail: elcamondobeach@gmail.com
Phone: +491751555847
Imprint: Independently published

www.ingramcontent.com/pod-product-compliance
Lightning Source LLC
Chambersburg PA
CBHW052307220526
45472CB00001B/14